UNHAPPY MEAL

STEPHANIE DANIEL and JOON YUN, M.D.

PALO ALTO INSTITUTE

A PALO ALTO INSTITUTE BOOK

PUBLISHED BY THE PALO ALTO INSTITUTE

PALO ALTO, CALIFORNIA

UNITED STATES OF AMERICA

[http://www.paloaltoinstitute.org]

COPYRIGHT © 2007 PALO ALTO INSTITUTE

ISBN 978-0-6151-4272-2

MANUFACTURED IN THE UNITED STATES OF AMERICA

COVER DESIGN BY SAM URTON

FIRST EDITION APRIL 2007

CONTENTS

1

THE WAY WE WERE

Walk around almost anywhere in the United States and the evidence is clearly visible—we as a nation are getting fatter. In 1960, just 13 percent of U.S. adults were obese. Today, 61 million people—nearly a third of all adults—are obese. The trend is similar worldwide—more than 300 million people are obese, a 50 percent jump since 1995. Conventional wisdom holds that rising rates of obesity come from people eating too much, eating food lacking in nutrition, and exercising too little.

But that sound bite fails to tell the whole story. The unsung culprit may very well be a condition we all deal with nearly every day—chronic stress. To understand why chronic stress leads to weight gain, we have to travel back in time a hundred thousand years.

The primary goal back then was survival. Every day, prehistoric humans had two main goals—to eat, and to not be eaten. Nature not only endowed us with the acute stress response to cope with encounters involving predators or prey, it also gave us a way to cope with more enduring ecologic challenges—the chronic stress response.

For instance, when resources became scarce, as might happen when winter approached or competition increased, the chronic stress response kicked in. Among other things, this response controlled the way the body managed its energy balance. Metabolism slowed and food-seeking behavior increased, as hoarding extra calories served the better part of prudence. When triggered for the right reasons, putting on a little extra fat made good Darwinian sense—doing so improved the chances for survival.

Nowadays, thanks to advances in modern agriculture, most of us in the developed world have little concern about running out of food. Unfortunately, although our lifestyles have evolved over the past hundred thousand years, our bodies have not. Chronic stress still triggers the same response it did way back when—although the chronic stress now comes about for reasons unrelated to concerns about the source of our next meal. We brood as we sit in traffic jams. We worry about financial troubles. We struggle with a lack of sleep. We fret when we read or watch news of death and destruction caused by war and natural disasters. All of these factors lead to our stress responses preparing our bodies for emergency survival mode.

So here is where evolution is failing us. We are chronically stressed despite the fact that we have an abundant supply of food. But the factory setting of our chronic stress response makes our bodies conserve energy, making us more metabolically efficient or more hungry in a mistaken anticipation of impending scarcity. It should come as no surprise that obesity in the U.S. has reached epidemic proportions. A growing body of evidence suggests that chronic stress may indeed play a role in our path to obesity.

One notable study found that women who slept 5 hours or less a night were 32 percent more likely to gain a significant amount of weight—33 pounds or more—than women who slept 7 hours a night. Both groups of women ate and exercised roughly the same amount. One possible explanation for this finding is that the women who slept less felt more stressed, contributing to their weight gain. Prednisone, a pharmaceutical version of a natural stress hormone, often leads to weight gain if taken chronically. Still another study found that children of parents who are strict disciplinarians are much more likely to become fat by the first grade, possibly due to authoritarian parenting which may trigger the children's chronic stress response and lead to weight gain.

Most of us know someone who quit smoking and subsequently gained a lot of weight. We might figure that the extra pounds simply came from the extra calories of food that our friend consumed as a substitute for cigarettes. However, when a smoker quits, the lack of nicotine triggers the body's stress response because the addiction to and craving for nicotine still exists. Then the metabolism slows, and the pounds start to pile on. A recent study showed that smokers who attempted to quit while taking antidepressants, which can also reduce anxiety, gained less weight than those smokers who did not take antidepressants.

We all know that in the long run, diets largely do not succeed in keeping the weight off. Eating less food and taking in fewer calories definitely lead to a reduction in weight in the short run. However, dieting may mistakenly suggest a scarcity of resources in the environment and may inadvertently even add to the chronic stress response. If caloric intake is reduced without the underlying stress being reduced, the body may become further predisposed towards hoarding calories. Consequently, once someone on a diet becomes satisfied with the amount of weight lost, and he or she resumes eating his or her usual foods, the tendency towards caloric hoarding can easily lead to a rebound gain in weight.

The link between chronic stress and weight gain is potentially life-threatening because the health implications of each condition are enormous. Interestingly, the list of chronic diseases to which stress reportedly contributes bears close similarity to the list of diseases associated with obesity: diabetes, heart disease, infection, lipid abnormalities, gout, behavioral disorders, stroke, depression, inflammation, sleep apnea, high blood pressure, infertility, and cancer. We believe that this apparent coincidence may arise in part from the significant contribution of chronic stress to the development of obesity.

Conversely, relieving chronic stress has enormous benefits. When we spend 30 minutes working out on the treadmill or the exercise bicycle, we are often disappointed that we've burned fewer calories than we hoped. Yet the significant weight loss accompanying such exercise suggests that the benefits of exercise may not be derived only through the burning of calories. Indeed, even a small amount of exercise can help us stay trim or lose more weight than we might think—when we exercise, we also relieve chronic stress and reverse some of the stress response already triggered in our bodies such as hoarding calories and excessive feelings of hunger. People who practice yoga regularly gain less weight over time than those who do not. We believe these benefits can be partly attributed to yoga's ability to relieve stress.

Exercise is terrific for reducing stress. So is improving our work and personal lifestyles and having better relationships with our family, friends, co-workers, neighbors, and even our enemies. Paying less attention to negative news in the media might help too. But is that enough?

2

SECONDHAND STRESS

In this book, we offer a novel theory that the food we eat is a significant, previously-unrecognized independent source of chronic stress—that a lot of the food we eat as part of the modern diet is itself stressed, and our body becomes stressed when we eat stressed foods.

With each meal, we take in more than just calories, protein, fats, and carbohydrates. We also absorb information about where the food came from and how it was raised, harvested, transported, and prepared. If our food faced stressful conditions along the way, it undergoes change. Our bodies then interpret this change as if we had undergone the stress ourselves. The stress we sense from the food chain may signal our bodies to store calories for what we perceive to portend challenging times ahead.

Nearly all plants and animals domesticated for human consumption are raised, processed, transported, stored, prepared, and consumed under highly unnatural, stressful conditions. For

example, salmon have gone through a similar progression. Salmon
have been part of the human diet for thousands of years.
Throughout history, hunter-gatherer societies caught wild salmon in
their native habitat, often in rivers and streams where they returned
to spawn. With the growing popularity of salmon over the last half
century, large commercial enterprises started raising salmon in
oceanic farms, known in the industry as aquaculture, to meet the
increasing demand by consumers. Farmed salmon live in higher-
density habitats, consume unnatural diets, have less room to roam,
and in general bear witness to a raft of unnatural, stressful
conditions, as compared to their wild counterparts.

It has become increasingly apparent that the cumulative
stress experience of animals and plants is encoded and embedded
throughout their bodies. While the source of chronic stress may
vary—unfavorable weather, infection or harsh husbandry
conditions—it becomes encoded in similar ways. For instance,
prolonged episodes of any type of stress in childhood are
permanently recorded in long bones as stress lines. Similarly, the
rings inside tree trunks, which help us determine the age of a tree,
actually represent records of ecologic stress endured by the tree.

The variation of temperature, sunlight, and water that
accompanies the seasons represents the most common and important
stress that impacts trees. Favorable climates, featuring adequate
moisture, long sunlight, and warm weather, produce wider spaces

between rings, whereas the rings themselves are created by the deceleration of growth. Each ring marks the passing of a year because it marks the passing of winter. Not surprisingly, rings are much more apparent in trees that grow in temperate climates, where seasons differ markedly in their extremes. Rings can also appear if the tree endures other forms of chronic stress, such as serious infection or trauma.

We believe that all plants and animals retain chronic stress in their body composition as certain types of fats and sugars, which then end up on our plate. Farmed fish and livestock that are raised in the confined, stressful conditions described above have different fat profiles—manifested in higher levels of saturated fat and a higher ratio of omega-6 to omega-3 fatty acids—as compared to wild fish.

Scientific research has shown that an increased intake of saturated fats may lead to negative effects on our health. Mounting data now also suggests that an elevated ratio of specific polyunsaturated long-chain fatty acids in our diet, specifically omega-6 to omega-3, portends future health problems. The ratio of omega-6 to omega-3 fatty acids in nature is presumed to have existed in the range of 1:1 to 3:1 prior to the development of agriculture. In modern-day Western diets, this ratio has deteriorated to 15:1 or even 30:1. Whereas a higher proportion of omega-3 fatty acids suppresses inflammation, a higher proportion of omega-6 fatty acids promotes it. This link is important because inflammation is a major risk factor for developing cardiovascular disease, cancer, and immune-mediated disease.

On the other hand, plants produce more simple sugars in their fruits when they experience chronic stress, most commonly due to oxidative factors. When we consume these simple sugars, whether in fruits or through manufacturing processes, they contribute to health problems very similar to those associated with unhealthy fats or chronic stress.

Only now have we begun to understand how these unhealthy fats and sugars can cause changes in our feeding behavior, alter our metabolism, and affect our tendencies towards particular illnesses. Evidence increasingly suggests that fats and sugars possess direct molecular signaling properties and can regulate biochemical and cell functions. Fats and sugars can directly target the brain and influence behavior.

Furthermore, fats and sugars can attach themselves to genes and proteins, the building blocks of life, and can influence their functions. In some cases, those altered biologic pathways can produce the kinds of behavioral and physiologic changes commonly observed in diseases associated with stress.

Fortunately, eating foods that have not undergone stressful experiences may provide health benefits potentially linked to reducing any ongoing stress response. For example, extra virgin olive oil requires production from just-pressed olives. Studies have shown that extra virgin olive oil has anti-inflammatory and heart-protective properties that its "regular" counterpart does not. Every criterion defining the extra virgin state also happens to reflect a reduction of chronic stress in the olive. For instance, extra virgin olive oil uses olives grown on trees that have escaped situations of disease and drought. Conversely, a protracted delay between picking and processing may increase chronic stress to the olive itself.

Indeed, whether from an animal or a plant, flesh may continue to undergo both organic and oxidative stress, even after being separated from the organism. Changes in color and taste bear evidence of this process. Eating fresh food likely imparts less stress to the consumer, since foods may accumulate stress following extensive transport, processing, handling, and preparation for cooking. Parceling out meat immediately following slaughter minimizes microbial contamination and dehydration, both of which may otherwise confer additional stress. The shorter the time from harvest to ingestion, the less stress foods may convey.

Vegetables, the non-reproductive parts of plants—that is, everything but the flowers and fruits—comprise one class of foods that generally appears to harbor less stress. Examples include stems, leaves, and roots. Unlike animals, plants generally do not depend on the presence of a particular aspect of these parts in order to function properly. A plant can suffer injury to multiple trunks or stems but continue to thrive. Because there is less at stake with the loss of any particular part, the stress response of any one part is less likely to be robust. As a result, any individual component of a plant is effectively less likely to "contain" indicators of stress. Consumption of roots, stems, and leaves may thus convey less stress to the consumer and lower the risk of stress-mediated disease. We believe that the inclusion of properly harvested plants may constitute the first step in developing a low-stress diet for our modern times.

Interest in healthy food has expanded over the last decade with the rise of many movements, including, but not limited to, locally-raised foods, organic foods, "slow foods", vegetarianism, raw foods, natural foods, and free-range meats. Each of these movements claims to offer health benefits that stem from its own specific philosophy. Rather than seeing them as independent, competing concepts, we believe that our low-stress foods theory is the unifying paradigm that links them under a common umbrella.

In the ensuing chapters, we first discuss the stress levels embedded in a variety of different food groups in more detail. The second half of this book provides suggestions to help you cut down on stress consumption by making different choices about the foods you eat, and by providing a list of resources, food stores, restaurants, and websites that help you access low-stress foods. In addition, we will delve into possible future strategies for making changes in our systems of food production to minimize the undesirable stress in our daily diet.

The implications are potentially significant. As mentioned previously, chronic stress is increasingly cited as a contributing factor in virtually all modern diseases, including heart disease, behavioral disorders, depression, auto-immune disease, gastrointestinal conditions, infertility, gout, infection, inflammatory conditions, pulmonary diseases, kidney diseases, and even cancer. Therefore, the consumption of a stressed diet may play a role in virtually all forms of chronic disease. These ideas may herald the birth of a brand new cottage industry—low-stress or stress-free foods—that may guide the cultivation, distribution, and consumption of food in the future. Radical social change might ensue as the food economy transforms.

Our bodies are designed to use food not only for nutrition, but also for information about the world around us. And like the negative headlines that populate today's media, our food may mislead us into thinking that we exist in a world of scarce resources, even though we are entering a time of unprecedented prosperity. This insight may represent the first step in enabling us to recognize the role that better food can play in mental and physical health. After reading this book, you may never look in your refrigerator or at your plate the same way again.

Which brings us to our first point of consideration—that all-American repast, the steak dinner.

3

DON'T HAVE A COW
(AT LEAST NOT A STRESSED ONE)

When we sit down for a steak dinner at home or in a restaurant, we typically see a well-manicured slab, quietly biding its time on the plate until we see fit to apply knife and fork. But that placid, pinkish façade may conceal a tortured upbringing.

Much of the modern beef industry has sprung up according to the model of mass production that came with industrialization. The ability to generate ever greater quantities of beef at decreasing prices led to an increasing appetite for beef on the part of the public. In order to keep up with this increasing demand, the beef industry has had to adopt methods to keep costs low and production high. Many of these practices have increased the levels of stress experienced by the animals.

For example, steers, or castrated male cattle, can be brought to market more quickly than untouched bulls, as the accumulation of fat occurs more quickly following castration. Consequently, within a few days of birth, male calves are castrated, frequently by means of surgery and without the use of anesthetic. Studies have measured the stress hormone cortisol in the blood of calves, and have shown that these indicators of stress increase following castration, particularly with the use of surgery. Around the same time, calves' horns may be removed by using a hot iron to cauterize the skin, creating a wound that often becomes susceptible to infestation by fly larvae.

In addition, calves are separated, or weaned, from their mothers in an abrupt fashion around the age of six months—an age earlier than would be the case in nature. Such calves become agitated and vocalize more, but eat and sleep less. Studies involving many species throughout nature have shown that separating offspring from their mothers imparts significant stress to the young. In the case of calves, premature separation from their mothers has been shown to increase the risk of respiratory illness, viral and parasitic infections, and even death in the young. Before their first year of life ends, these calves may experience as much stress as their wild counterparts may undergo in a lifetime. But their ordeal has only just begun.

Most cattle raised in the United States have to withstand at least two protracted periods of travel. First, they are rousted from the cow-calf farm and taken to the feedlot to be fattened. Then, once they become suitable for market, they are taken to the slaughterhouse. Intervening events such as auctions only further increase the time spent in transport.

Ground transportation and a need to keep costs low encourage sequestration of cattle in claustrophobic spaces, a concept referred to as "high stocking density." There the cattle must endure vehicle vibrations, noise, exhaust fumes, wind, and extreme temperatures, as well as a relative deprivation of food, water, and sleep. As expected, such practices lead to findings of stress such as increased heart rate and increased cortisol levels. The high stocking density also negatively impacts movement patterns and leads to increased risks of injury such as bruising.

Laboratory indicators of dehydration stress occur in animals that are on the road for even relatively short periods of time, ranging from roughly half a day to a day and a half. Even shorter transport times produce physical signs of dehydration, as well as disruption of normal feeding patterns that require several days to revert to normal. Policy does not mandate rest periods for cattle transported by truck, meaning that most animals have little respite during their journeys. Calves are especially affected by the stress from transport. Calves imported into North Dakota were found to have significantly higher rates of illness and death than those indigenous to the region.

A syndrome attributed to bacteria and viruses, bovine respiratory disease has been traditionally ascribed to the rigors of transport; indeed, the colloquial term for the condition is "shipping fever." It affects over 10 percent of animals and has been implicated in over half the cases of pre-market mortality among cattle. In addition, although 35 percent of feedlot steers received treatment for this illness, at the time of slaughter over two-thirds had lung pathology suggesting progression to pneumonia.

Upon reaching the feedlot, shelter is frequently minimal, as dust, mud, and animal waste accumulate in conjunction with exposure to elements ranging from high temperatures to wind and precipitation. Branding can add to the calves' stress. Although animals can also be identified by tagging the ears, or by generating wattle and earmarks by cutting pieces of skin around the neck and ears, branding still persists as the most commonly used practice to achieve this end. Whether accomplished through either the traditional direct application of a hot iron or by freezing, the use of branding clearly produces stress. Studies comparing the use of a sham, or non-heated brand, to an actual heated or frozen brand showed increases in several measures of stress in the branded group, including elevated blood stress hormone levels, heart rates, escape-avoidance reactions, and other behaviors associated with pain.

Because most cattle spend the first six months of their lives at a cow-calf farm grazing on open pasture, the experience of handling itself can prove extremely stressful. The intensity of handling can range from mild to aversive, with practices such as roping, shouting, hitting, tail twisting, and shocking with an electrical prod. Increased heart rates and excessive movement result from hearing shouts, a response that endures for several days or more. Blood stress hormone levels on average are two-thirds higher in those cattle handled roughly, and such animals also show signs of susceptibility to bruising. Techniques used to restrain cattle also invoke stress responses, ranging from heart rate increases with mild restraint to responses akin to those seen with branding with more intense restraints such as squeeze chutes.

The animals are kept at the feedlot until they reach their desired market weight. This process typically takes anywhere from four months to one year, and requires an average daily weight gain of 3 pounds. The rapid and progressive weight accumulation leads to physical stress on the legs, producing cartilage damage and pain, compounded by a lack of exercise due to cramped quarters.

In order to achieve the requisite growth required to bring animals to market, a potpourri of artificial growth promoters is administered through both ingestion and injection. One such component of this regimen is antibiotics. Animals routinely receive antibiotics to prevent illness and to encourage growth. Surveys show that over 50 percent of feedlots give antibiotics as standard practice upon receipt of animals, and nearly all gave them at some point during the course of an animal's stay. The majority of these feedlots incorporate antibiotics into feed and water. The use of these antibiotics has led to the development of strains of infectious bacteria which are multiply resistant to various antibiotics, an increasing source of stress and disease.

Hormones make up another part of the prescription for growth. The incentive to use hormones comes from a significant return on investment—20 to 50 additional pounds of weight per cattle can be achieved from a single hormonal implant costing one to two dollars. Nearly all cattle receive hormone implants, and some more than a single time. These hormones include estrogens, testosterone, and synthetic steroids. A lack of understanding remains as to how these agents act, given their protean influence. However, since the administration of these hormones is not physiologic, intuition suggests that this disruption of endocrine homeostasis likely causes stress.

Of course, diet represents the foundation for achieving growth targets. However, animals in feedlots do not partake of a natural cattle diet, which consists of roughage such as grass, plants, and shrubs. Instead, roughage makes up less than 10 percent of a standard feedlot diet, with the majority comprised of readily fermentable, starchy, and low-fiber carbohydrate-laden grains such as wheat and corn, as well as byproducts of corn grown from genetically modified plants.

Although this feed composition provides high levels of energy that contribute to rapid weight gain, the lack of fiber produces stress and strain on the gastrointestinal tract and the overall metabolism of the animal. Indeed, if the feed itself is comprised of stressed grains, one can envision a chain reaction as stress signals ripple through the web.

Digestive problems such as bloat have been reported to affect nearly 2 percent of all cattle, whereas acidosis has become so pervasive that antibiotic usage to maintain acidosis prevalence of less than 20 percent is considered a success. Lameness due to impaired blood circulation to the hooves is on the rise and also constitutes a direct consequence of feedlot practices; increased stomach acidity from the low-fiber high-energy diet enhances the absorption of toxins into the bloodstream.

Stress also plays a role in the slaughterhouse. While the well-being of animals is taken into consideration, economic factors likely also play a role, as an adrenaline surge prior to dispatch results in a darker, less tasty cut of meat. The animals that yield such meat are referred to as "dark cutters."

Until the beginning of this millennium, lax administration of anesthesia often meant that animals remained conscious even as they underwent slaughter. At that time, revisions to the slaughtering process were made in an attempt to minimize potential distress and suffering on the part of the animal. Even then, the resultant carcass emerges caked with manure and bacteria, necessitating passage of the body through a hot steam cabinet, followed by a spray treatment with an antimicrobial solution, and finishing with irradiation of the meat prior to its preparation for sale.

The odyssey from calf to plate appears fraught with chronic stress. There is increasing evidence that this pilgrimage has yielded untoward effects on the meat itself. The beef now carries the experience of stress within it, and will affect the consumer—us—accordingly. As discussed in the previous chapter, even though the sources of chronic stress may differ, the same pattern of abnormal lipid profiles emerges, showcasing relatively high levels of saturated fats and omega-6 fatty acids.

When raised on a low-fiber high-energy diet and held in close captivity, cattle yield beef that demonstrates both higher saturated fat content as well as a higher omega-6 to omega-3 fatty acid ratio, as compared to beef from animals allowed to subsist on their native diet of roughage while roaming open pastures, free from chemical interventions. In controlled studies, cattle fed diets of varying composition yielded the lowest levels of saturated fat in their meat when their diet consisted purely of grass. Levels of saturated fat increased as the dietary component of grass was reduced and a component based on a grain concentrate was increased.

It would appear that the stress experienced by these animals does translate to changes in their meat, which in turn produces potentially harmful effects when eaten. To reiterate, diseases associated with the consumption of a diet high in saturated fats or certain omega fatty acid ratios are virtually identical to the diseases found in conjunction with chronic stress. We suggest that these dietary signals communicate stress to consumers, whose bodies then recapitulate the stress response.

4

MILKING IT
(FOR ALL IT'S WORTH)

Since the time of their initial domestication in the Neolithic era, cows have served as a source of milk. Up until the middle of the nineteenth century, consumption of milk products revolved around the family-owned cow. However, the development of pasteurization changed everything. When this means of preservation was combined with an increased knowledge of selective breeding, refrigerated means of transport, and automated milking and bottling machines, the dairy industry began to take shape.

Not until the latter half of this past century, however, did true industrialization in the form of mechanization emerge. In the past two decades, while the number of farms with dairy cows has gone from well over 300,000 to just over 100,000, the overall production of milk has increased more than 30 percent. One factor explaining this finding involves an increase in herd size. Over that same period, the number of dairy farms with more than 100 animals in their herd nearly doubled, with well over 1,000 dairy farms with herd sizes numbering 1,000 or greater by 2004.

Like their meat-producing counterparts, dairy farms use techniques to wring the greatest production out of the lowest cost. Three out of four dairy cows never graze on pasture, and many do not have access to the outdoors. They receive low-fiber high-energy grain-based feed in conjunction with growth hormones and antibiotics, yielding a tendency to develop lameness. If subjected to prodding, shouting, tail-twisting, and hitting, they show physical signs of stress each time they witness a handler who has previously subjected them to such behavior. They also undergo dehorning and incur both pain and an increased infection risk as a result.

Most female calves born on dairy farms spend their entire lives on a particular farm and do not suffer the stress of frequent transport. Despite evidence showing that later separation may result in greater milk production, improved health, and fewer behavioral problems, they undergo separation from their mother at an earlier age than would occur in nature, with less than 10 percent allowed to nurse longer than one day after birth. Feedings following separation occur twice a day, a lower frequency than would be the case for regular nursing. Studies show that calves provided access to a continuous supply of milk consumed nearly twice as much and gained over 63 percent more weight than calves fed on a restricted schedule.

Calves are often kept in isolation from each other in crates until they are at least 5 weeks old. Most farms also restrict contact between calves and adult cattle, all in a bid to reduce transmission of infectious disease. Studies have demonstrated a benefit from housing calves in groups, with decreased exhibition of stress-induced behaviors such as vocalizing, rutting, and excessive licking. In addition, calves housed in crates which lacked adequate space showed suppression of the immune system, an indicator of stress.

In addition to dehorning, dairy calves undergo tail docking. This procedure, which involves amputation of a portion of the tail, is performed for presumed reasons of hygiene. The most frequent techniques deploy either a rubber ring around the tail to cut off blood supply, or a heated docking iron to simultaneously cut and cauterize. Either approach infrequently involves the use of anesthesia. In addition to inflicting short-term pain, the procedure prohibits the cows from using their tails for communication. It also curtails their ability to ward off flying insects, exposing the cows to more episodes of biting and ongoing stress. In addition, certain cows suffer chronic pain in similar fashion to the phantom limb pain experienced by human amputees.

The housing experienced by dairy cows varies by geographic region and may range from pastures to earthen corrals (dry lots), to bedded pens (straw yards), to barns with open cubicles (free stalls), to barns with tether cubicles (tie stalls). Over half of dairy cows live in tie stalls. The tie stall represents the most space-efficient but also the most restrictive of these arrangements in terms of physical movement. Studies have shown that teat and mammary infections occur more frequently in cows kept in tie stalls as compared to those kept in free stalls or straw yards. The use of tie stalls is also associated with a higher incidence of bloat, as well as that of hoof and leg disorders. Those cows kept in tie stalls with limited access to the outdoors experience more lameness, more skin injuries around the neck, and more joint injuries as compared to those cows with the ability to engage in regular exercise. Cows housed on concrete floors have difficulty standing up and lying down, and 80 percent of such cows have at least one form of hoof disorder. Those cows restrained four or more hours a day spent more time lying down and engaged in more grooming behaviors once released.

Even open dry lots which allow for relative freedom of movement can inflict stress on cows through the consequences of elemental exposure. Heavy rains can lead to the formation of mud in conjunction with manure. The mud precludes freedom of movement, access to food, and the ability to lie down. It also provides a haven for bacteria, again increasing the risk of lameness and inflammation of the teats, also known as mastitis. The risk of a particular hoof disorder is far lower in the context of pasture, which allows for free drainage and a lower propensity for mud formation.

This risk remains reduced even in the case of pasture combined with dry lots when compared to dry lots alone.

Cows that graze on pasture engage in fewer aggressive interactions and are more likely to behave in concert in terms of eating and sleeping with other cows. Cows that graze on pasture and have access to their natural diet of grass show a lower prevalence of virtually all diseases found in cows. Unfortunately, the number of dairy farms with access to pasture continues to decline; over a five-year period from 1996 to 2001 the number of dairy farms with no access to pasture increased from 50 percent to just over 75 percent of all farms.

Dairy cows are subjected to unnatural lighting conditions. The use of increased light exposure to suppress melatonin, a hormone produced in the pineal gland, delays the onset of the dry period, when milk production stops. During lactation, increasing the period of light exposure to 16 hours a day yields an additional 4 pounds of milk per day on average. During the dry period, reversing the schedule so that cows receive 16 hours of darkness and only 8 hours of light increases milk production by as much as 6 pounds per day during the next lactation. However, such deviance from normal sleep-wake schedules is well known to induce stress in many animals.

Seventy percent of dairy cows are milked in a parlor system, characterized by large holding pens that hold the cows in queue for milking. Standing for hours in close quarters on unnatural surfaces such as the concrete floors of these pens increases the cows' susceptibility to lameness. Cows new to the milking process and subjected to close interaction with either unfamiliar human handlers or an unfamiliar environment show signs of stress, such as a higher heart rate and increased cortisol levels. Milking multiple times a day has been shown to increase production yield, but also exposes the cows to more handling stress.

Most large dairy operations use artificial insemination for impregnation to start the process of milk production. For this purpose, cows are often held in a stall for prolonged periods of time and have little contact with other cows. They are made to face a wall and are unable to move around, lie down, or lick themselves. They also have no direct access to food and water.

Insemination seeks to minimize the time between births, or calving interval, by maximizing the time during which the cow produces milk. The average calving interval is typically a little over thirteen months, and less than 5 percent of all dairy operations have a calving interval longer than sixteen months. Dairy cows typically only spend 60 days out of a year "dry", or not producing milk. They typically undergo a gestation, or pregnancy period, of nine months, and then undergo insemination again within three months of giving birth.

In addition, artificial insemination with semen from bulls with favorable characteristics has permitted the selective breeding of cows specific for their ability to produce milk. Over the past fifteen years, the volume of milk production has increased 20 percent. Such cows have also increased in average size, increasing their susceptibility to problems such as lameness and mastitis, and making the smaller existing enclosures even more limiting in terms of movement. Selective breeding has also produced animals with higher rates of mammary, digestive, locomotive, and respiratory disease.

Growth hormone administration to dairy cows deserves particular mention. Around one-fourth of all dairy cows in the United States receive bovine somatotropin, also known as bovine growth hormone, despite the banning of its use in both Canada and the European Union out of safety concerns. Although the hormone increases milk production by an average of 14 percent a day, side effects can include reduced fertility, increased frequency of ovarian cysts, mastitis, increased body temperature, indigestion, bloat, diarrhea, anorexia, enlarged hocks, foot lesions, and injection site reactions. The increased risk for mastitis necessitates more frequent use of antibiotics and its attendant consequences. The increase in body temperature can lead to a lower tolerance of heat and a greater vulnerability to heat stress.

Ultimately, however, the key finding may simply be that the milk from cows raised on pasture contains up to five times more conjugated linoleic acid, an omega-3 fatty acid with anti-inflammatory properties, than milk from cows raised on high-energy grain feed. The presence of a stressed fat profile in milk may have enabled the cow to effectively instruct her calves to properly prepare for current and future exigencies. Drinking such milk, especially when transported far from its source, may lead to our own bodies inappropriately responding to these signals as if they legitimately reflected prevailing stress.

Indeed, even after milk leaves the cow, it may incorporate further degrees of stress on its way to our glasses. Most milk undergoes pasteurization, which involves heating the milk to high temperatures in order to achieve relative sterility, thereby extending its shelf life. In addition to pasteurization, most milk also undergoes homogenization, a process whereby the fat globules of cream become reduced to a smaller size, enabling them to achieve an even suspension throughout the milk and preventing them from separating out and floating to the surface. It remains unknown whether exposure of the biochemical components of milk to extreme conditions associated with pasteurization and homogenization imparts molecular stress. What is known is that pasteurization can affect the three-dimensional conformations of the proteins in milk. It can also destroy the activity of lactase, an enzyme contained in milk that assists in its metabolism, as well as vitamins and potentially beneficial bacteria.

Thus cows that live under conditions of low stress likely produce the same molecular indicator of contentment that we find in their meat-yielding counterparts—a signal that when ingested, can reduce our stress. On the other hand, dairy cows raised under stressful conditions are more likely to produce milk with high saturated fat levels and unfavorable fatty acid ratios.

5

FLAGRANT FOWL

Like the beef industry, the chicken meat industry has undergone consolidation into commercial conglomerates. Until the 1920s, most chickens were raised independently on family farms for local consumption and use. At that time, the so-called "broiler" chicken, intended for mass production and distribution, was developed in various regions, including the Delmarva Peninsula (Delaware, Maryland, Virginia), Georgia, Arkansas, and New England.

The early industry consisted of separately held entities of feed mills, hatcheries, farms, and processors. Within forty years, 90 percent of the broiler business came from vertically integrated entities. By the year 2005, chicken had become the single most consumed meat in the United States, nearly 98 percent of which constitutes the broiler variety.

In the 1920s, chicken came to market an average of 112 days following hatching. By the year 2005, this number had more than halved to 48 days—less than seven weeks after hatching. At the same time, the weight of the chicken brought to market has more than doubled from 2 1/2 pounds to just over 5 1/2 pounds. These changes have occurred through a combination of practices— selective breeding for enlarged breasts, administration of growth-promoting chemicals, and use of corn and soy in high caloric feed.

Selective breeding has led to chickens that can yield increasing amounts of breast meat. Unfortunately, the birds have also become too large for their limbs to support them. Gait abnormalities have been found in up to 90 percent of all birds, and up to half suffer from some form of leg deformity. By the age of six weeks, chickens spend anywhere from 76 to 86 percent of their time lying down. The rapid rates of growth contribute to respiratory disease, enlargement of the liver and spleen, accumulation of fluid in the abdomen, and enlargement of the heart, leading to acute death syndrome from arrhythmias.

Chickens are housed in warehouse-like sheds termed "grower houses", which provide an average of 130 square inches per bird. This amount of space is less than what is required for a typical bird at rest and reduces the possibility of normal behaviors such as preening, foraging, and extending the wings. Accumulation of excrement can lead to high levels of ammonia, which increases the chickens' susceptibility to respiratory illnesses and blindness. Ammonia levels pose a particular issue during winters, when they rise due to a need to limit ventilation to maintain adequate heating. Although arsenic is still routinely used as an appetite stimulant to increase feeding, the role of antibiotics in the poultry industry has shifted from that of a growth promoter and a standard component of feed to that of use on an as-needed basis.

When broiler chickens reach 45 days of age, they undergo crating for transport to slaughter. People responsible for crating the animals do so at a rate of 1,000 to 1,500 birds per hour, resulting in injuries such as fractures and dislocations of hips, legs and wings, as well as internal bleeding. Studies have shown that chickens exhibit high levels of stress hormones during transport. Common ailments during transport include hypothermia, hyperthermia, and heart failure.

Upon arrival at the slaughterhouse, the chickens' legs undergo shackling, producing additional fractures and dislocations. The federal Humane Methods of Slaughter Act does not apply to poultry, meaning that chickens may remain aware during the course of their slaughter. One study found that nearly a quarter of all chickens remained conscious at the time of immersion into scalding water to remove their feathers. The meat from chickens subjected to these practices has a lower ratio of omega-3 fatty acids to omega-6 fatty acids than their free-range counterparts—the same unhealthy profile we see in other farmed meats grown under stressful conditions, and the same profile associated with many stress-related diseases in humans that consume them.

The eggs of chickens experience the same fate as the hens that laid them. In the wild, hens spend most of their time walking around foraging, pecking, scratching at the ground, and bathing in dust. They perch at rest, and typically search out nesting places in secluded locations enclosed by vegetation and contours in the ground. In contrast, 95 percent of the 350 million egg-laying hens in the United States are kept in the poultry counterpart of the tie stall, the battery cage.

Battery cages consist of stacked wire cages with sloped floors which typically house anywhere from 3 to 10 hens. The space per chicken amounts to 61 square inches on average—less than the size of a sheet of paper—and can be as little as 48 square inches. For purposes of comparison, studies have shown that hens occupy an average of 236 square inches at rest and 787 square inches to extend their wings. Although the European Union has proposed a phase-out of the battery cage arrangement by 2012, the United Egg Producers, an American trade union, has only made a commitment thus far to increasing the size allotment to 67 square inches—an upgrade of 7 square inches.

As expected, these confines produce both acute and chronic stress. Thirst and water retention represent classic signatures of stress—the desire to hoard water in anticipation of challenging times. Studies have shown that hens housed in battery cages took five times longer to drink and drank more frequently than their so-called free-range counterparts, suggesting that caged birds are experiencing greater stress. The usual 554 square inches of restricted space are insufficient to meet the hens' requirements for adequate social spacing. In the face of crowding, the normally cohesive social structure of hens disintegrates, leading to increased manifestation of aggressive behaviors.

To minimize injury, the hens' beaks are often trimmed, a traumatic procedure involving cutting and cautery first performed at 6 days of age and again between 7 to 11 weeks of age to curtail regrowth. Since the procedure is primarily done without anesthesia, it often leads to acute and chronic pain due to the extensive nerve supply of the beak, and is worsened further by the formation of neuromas, bundles of nerve tissue that form in the healed stump of the beak. Studies have shown disturbances in sleep, eating, grooming, and social behavior following trimming, as well as increases in stress hormone levels and reduced body weight due to depressed feed consumption. These manifestations of stress may arise not only from the procedure, but also from the loss of beak function, as the beak serves a number of grasping and manipulating functions with respect to feeding, nesting, drinking, preening, and defense.

Caged hens also frequently develop fatty liver hemorrhagic syndrome. This syndrome appears to arise from a combination of a lack of exercise, confinement-induced stress, and consumption of high-energy grain-based feeds. It features the deposition of large amounts of fat in the liver, leading ultimately to liver rupture.

Despite the increased stress suffered by the hens, the battery cage concept carries significant economic advantages. High-density housing lowers costs and facilitates other means to compel increased egg production. One such mechanism to achieve this objective involves forced molting.

Molting, the period when chickens exchange old feathers for new, occurs after a period of egg production and must conclude before a new egg-laying cycle can occur. In the wild, this period lasts approximately 16 weeks. However, both by depriving the hens of food for up to 12 days and water for up to 3 days, and by instituting constant artificial light exposure for 7 days, egg producers have shortened this hiatus to a period of only 8 weeks.

Although forced molting means more rapid turnover between egg-laying cycles and higher levels of egg production, studies have shown evidence of chronic stress, particularly in the form of reduced immunity. Hens undergoing forced molting had significantly lower numbers of circulating lymphocytes, a type of white blood cell that is involved in immunity, as well as reduced delayed-type hypersensitivity, a measure of immunologic responsiveness.

Any illness contracted by the hens during this period typically compels administration of antibiotics. Antibiotics can disrupt the hens' natural intestinal bacteria and make them more susceptible to disease, often with the result of producing

contaminated eggs. Even without the use of antibiotics, studies have

shown that chronic exposure to artificial light itself increases

colonization by Salmonella bacteria. As mentioned previously,

exposure to abnormal patterns of light can induce physiologic stress

and suppress the immune system of many species.

Egg production with these techniques reaches an average of

260 eggs per hen per year, roughly ten times as many as the wild

ancestor of the modern hen, the Red Junglefowl, would lay in a

year—25. This artificially high level of egg production also affects

the health of hens. Bone weakness secondary to osteoporosis, from

the increased calcium demand needed to form the shells and a lack

of exercise, affects nearly 90 percent of all caged hens, with

fractures prior to transport affecting one-sixth of all hens. Uterine

prolapse, or the expulsion of the uterus outside the body cavity of

the hen, can also occur through a combination of the frequency of

egg-laying and the size of the eggs laid—far larger than seen

historically due to the use of high-energy grain-based feeds.

Various studies have shown that eggs produced by hens

raised in the battery-cage environment have lower levels of the

antioxidants vitamin A, vitamin E, and beta-carotene, as well as

higher levels of cholesterol, than eggs taken from so-called free-

range hens. One study showed that eggs from free-range hens had

triple the levels of the anti-inflammatory omega-3 fatty acid found in hens raised in battery cages on a commercial diet. Other studies have shown elevation of saturated fat content in eggs laid by hens held in battery cages or fed unnatural diets.

Any perceived health risks popularly ascribed to eggs may not be intrinsic to the egg in and of itself, but rather may arise as a consequence of production by stressed hens. A hen that lives a difficult existence will attempt to "teach" its offspring—its eggs—to prepare for stressful conditions by encoding this knowledge in the yolk that the embryonic chick will consume. By eating such eggs, we may end up inadvertently intercepting these stress signals and assuming the disposition of the distressed hens.

Even as recently as a few decades ago, eating a fish- or plant-based diet may have served as a way to circumvent these concerns. Skirting the issues imposed by modern meat and poultry processing practices may explain the relative longevity of such ethnicities as Okinawans, who use wild fish as a staple of their diet. However, modern technology has managed to systematically permeate this food with messages of chronic stress as well. Amongst fish, the story of salmon presents a particularly vivid example of this process at work.

6

UP THE CREEK

Although salmon constitute a staple of the human diet in many regions of the world, such as Japan, Scandinavia, and Russia, mass consumption of this fish in the United States represents a relatively recent phenomenon. Production has gone from 50,000 metric tons per year two decades ago to well over 1,000,000 metric tons per year today. In order to accommodate this demand, the predominant source of salmon has shifted from that of commercial fishing to that of farming.

The idea of raising salmon broods in areas of the ocean restricted by netting was conceived as part of a research initiative to replenish depleted salmon runs in the northeastern part of the country. Soon adapted for commercial purposes, the practice of farming first appeared in Northern Europe and then spread to Chile and British Columbia. Individual farms now produce close to 9,000 tons of farmed salmon on an annual basis, and global conglomerates control syndicates of farms. Farmed salmon is less expensive than its wild counterpart, and now accounts for 70 percent of the global salmon supply. Nearly all farmed salmon in the United States has its origins in species found in the Atlantic, as wild Atlantic salmon themselves have become endangered and are no longer actively fished. Salmon found in the Pacific Ocean represent one of five species and remain actively fished.

Wild salmon migrate from fresh water to the ocean following birth and return to the ocean to spawn. In contrast, the life of farmed salmon begins with the harvesting of eggs from a mature female salmon. Following prescreening for disease and disinfection with chemicals, the eggs are incubated until the time of hatching. The time from initial incubation to hatching typically takes 6 to 7 weeks. The hatchlings then spend an additional 20 to 30 days growing. They then undergo handling and grading for size and uniformity before being transferred to freshwater rearing tanks.

The next 12 to 18 months are then spent growing to a mature weight of about 60 grams. At that time they are displaced once again to large open salt water sea cages in the ocean, where they remain for the next 1 to 2 years until they reach market size. These cages typically constitute large steel or plastic mesh bags tethered to the ocean floor, holding up to 50,000 fish in a space measuring 30 square meters with a depth of 20 meters. Space comes at a premium; each adult salmon swims in the equivalent of a bathtub of water. Frequent trauma from rubbing up against the sides of the cage and each other leads to injury to gills and fins.

Considering the degree of activity required of wild salmon to carry out their responsibility to perpetuate the species—namely, swimming upstream to spawn— confinement likely affects the physical well-being of salmon more than it would affect the average species, as it interferes with their natural behavioral programming. Indeed, mortality on many farms can range as high as 30 percent, and some farms can lose as many as 200,000 fish a year.

Due to the absence of a barrier protecting them from the surrounding aquatic environment, fish in sea cages remain exposed to ongoing sources of stress in the form of agents of infection and waste contamination, with little option for avoidance or defense due to their physical confinement. Infectious salmon anemia, a viral illness characterized by blanching of the gills, swelling of the liver, and internal bleeding, may necessitate wholesale slaughter to prevent spread of the disease. In the span of two years alone (1998-1999), eight million fish had to be sacrificed in Scotland. Kudoa, another parasite, softens the muscle of salmon post-mortem to a near-liquid consistency, making it commercially worthless. Undetectable prior to processing, kudoa affects 20 to 50 percent of salmon produced in British Columbia alone.

Even those infections that lend themselves to treatment may compromise the salmon further as the result of the treatment alone. Sea lice are small crustaceans that injure salmon through chewing, leading to either direct loss or increased susceptibility to bacterial infections. One study showed a 30,000-fold higher density of sea lice in one salmon farm as compared to the open ocean. Treatment of sea lice requires dousing the fish with such chemicals as organophosphates, pyrethoids, and hydrogen peroxide, themselves toxins and chemical irritants.

Bacterial contamination from waste exposure and crowding can lead to infection, termed furunculosis, as well as kidney and intestinal disease. Bacterial kidney disease alone accounts for nearly 10 percent of Pacific salmon farm loss. In order to control these risks, salmon farms typically use at least five different antibiotics in large quantities. In the year 2003 alone, farms in Chile used over 2,000 tons of antibiotics. Antibiotic exposure not only affects bacteria, but also the fish themselves, where agents such as oxytetracycline act as promoters of growth. Chronic exposure may lead to promotion of chronic stress.

Studies have shown depressed immune system function, a classic sign of chronic stress, in farmed salmon as compared to wild salmon. The handling and grading of salmon appears to invoke other proxies for stress such as elevated serum concentrations of lactate, glucose, and chloride, and depressed hemoglobin and hematocrit. Other witnessed signs of presumed chronic stress in these settings include behavioral changes such as spontaneous migration to one region of the cage and increased breathing activity.

Whereas wild salmon normally feed on insects, crayfish, and other crustaceans as part of a carnivorous diet, farmed salmon receive an unnatural diet composed of an artificially processed mixture of fish meal, fish oil, grains, vitamins, and minerals administered in pellet form. The pink color of farmed salmon must be endowed through the use of a synthetic pigment, canthaxanthin that is given as a supplement to their feed, in contrast the pink color of wild salmon arises naturally from the ingestion of krill. Concerns regarding a link between canthaxanthin and retinal damage has limited its use in Europe and necessitated the institution of labeling in the United States.

Not unlike cattle, farmed salmon reach their market size in an accelerated fashion. They typically do so after an average of 3 years of life, in contrast to wild salmon which typically require 7 years to reach the same point. However, prior to slaughter, they are starved for 7 to 10 days in order to minimize the risk of contamination during the gutting process. Slaughter itself involves a variety of traumatic approaches, including stunning with carbon dioxide, cutting the gills without anesthesia, and inducing suffocation either in plain air or on ice, the last of which sustains sensation for up to 15 minutes after removal from the water.

Again, the body compositions of wild and farmed salmon differ significantly. Farmed Atlantic salmon can harbor up to 70 percent more fat as compared to its wild Atlantic brethren, and almost 3 times as much fat as compared to wild Pacific or chum salmon. As previously noted, the factory setting in nature is to hoard calories under conditions of chronic stress, so the fattening seen in farmed salmon does not come as a surprise. Unfortunately, the chronic stress that precipitates these biologic changes in farmed salmon is biochemically encoded in their bodies. Farmed salmon typically has more than twice as much saturated fat than its wild counterpart. The ratio of omega-3 fatty acids to omega-6 fatty acids in wild Atlantic salmon is nearly 4 to 1, as opposed to farmed Atlantic salmon where the ratio is closer to 1 to 1. Eating farmed salmon may expose humans to these dietary components classically linked to many diseases associated with stress.

The imposition of stress can occur even in the last stages of processing prior to serving, as illustrated by the preparation of fish for sushi. Stale fish can be concealed in the form of spicy tuna rolls to obscure any betrayals of flavor. The rosy red hue of apparently fresh flesh may have come from treatment with carbon monoxide to bind hemoglobin. Flash freezing and sourcing from multiple vendors have replaced timely delivery of the catch from a known provider. For many sushi chefs, Japan remains the supplier of choice due to more progressive methods of preparation and richer sources of plankton feed. Most recently, a chef in Japan has investigated using acupuncture to anesthetize still-living fish prior to preparation. Although apparent economic benefits come from storing a great number of idle rather than active fish in the same amount of space, minimizing the stress to these fish may yield health benefits for ourselves as well.

All told, confinement, coupled with frequent handling and transport, unnatural diet, exposure to antibiotics and chemical disinfectants, as well as increased risks of disease and waste contamination, combined with an accelerated program of growth, leads to a situation not unlike that found with cattle and chickens, with similar alterations in body composition. Chronic stress appears to serve as the unifying factor in all of these instances.

7

LOOPY FRUITS

More so than animals, plants grown in the wild tend to diversify in the forms that they assume. In the absence of intervention, their characteristics in terms of size, color, and taste cannot be reliably predicted from generation to generation, which reduces their value as a food item. Fig trees may have represented the first plants cultivated for the purposes of food, found in the Jordan River Valley more than a millennium before staples such as wheat and barley became domesticated in the Middle East. Mutations in the ancient fig apparently produced sweetness of fruit accompanied by a loss of seeds, thereby compelling the participation of humans to allow the mutation to persist. They did so either by taking a cutting from a sterile tree and grafting it onto the base of another tree, termed a rootstock, or by planting the cutting directly into the ground, hoping for it to take root and grow. These practices are termed cultivation, and can lend themselves to not only survival, but also convenience.

One form of cultivation done today to ease harvesting involves grafting a cutting to a dwarf rootstock to create artificially dwarfed varieties of trees. Modern-day agriculture continues this reliance on cultivating a very small number of genetic variants, or monoculture. Monoculture differs from permaculture, or the way sustainable growth occurs in the wild, in that it can only exist within a relatively narrow set of environmental parameters without risking extinction. The planting of orchards, or the planting of a particular variety of plants without planting other varieties or species close by, constitutes one key practice of monoculture, as opposed to permaculture, where a variety of species grow in close proximity as they would in nature.

In order to keep this unnatural state of existence intact, other artificial processes must be instituted. Whereas plants grow in the wild according to the patterns of rainfall and terrain that will naturally support their growth, cultivation requires irrigation in order to overcome habitats such as desert or swampland that would normally not sustain the type of species under consideration. Pollination occurs by hand rather than by insects, birds, or the wind, as is the case in the wild. Chemical fertilizers, pesticides, and fungicides compensate for the relative inability of plants to adapt when uprooted from their native soil. More recently, direct genetic manipulation via the production of GMO (genetically modified organisms) has become an increasingly popular method to improve the hardiness of plants.

Yet despite the pampering given to the domesticated forms, the wild varieties of plants typically remain far more robust and impervious to stress, as evidenced by their thick density of growth. As late as the latter part of the nineteenth century, wild blackberries were considered a weed rather than a potential source for food.

As a result of these manipulations to improve survival combined with selective breeding to improve taste, those parts of cultivated plants that we eat typically depart significantly from those found with their wild cousins. Fruits simply represent the ripened reproductive organs of flowering plants, with variations in characteristics likely related to their mode of dispersal. Plants relying on distribution in the droppings of birds or animals likely gained characteristics that made them more favorable to ingestion.

Nonetheless, maximizing these features never comes at the expense of the primary objective of preserving the seed. For example, wild fruits typically contain large seeds, small amounts of fruit flesh, high quantities of fiber, and are relatively small in size. They tend to taste more sour, bitter, or even astringent, with a far lower sugar content than might be expected.

However, to fit the economics and taste preferences of mass consumption by humans, the efforts of cultivation have sought to exaggerate sweetness in fruit, as well as to minimize seed size or eliminate seeds completely. The goal here is to maximize the amount of fruit flesh available for consumption and to reduce the hassle involved with eating it. Consequently, most cultivated fruits end up significantly larger and lower in fiber content than would be the case in the wild.

Production of fruit for mass consumption has led to other measures that deviate from natural behaviors. Cultivated fruit trees may be forced to bloom and fruit on an annual basis, as opposed to a biennial basis as is the case with many varieties in the wild. When ripe, wild fruit naturally detaches itself from its stem. However, the harvest of cultivated fruit occurs prior to the time of its natural ripening, and often before it even reaches its stage of mature greenness. Ripe fruit cannot withstand the rigors of processing and transport, which often involve significant distances.

Furthermore, many fruits are grown away from their natural habitat in terms of soil, surrounding ecosystem, climate, and season. Chemicals may be used to coerce detachment in conjunction with mechanical harvesting. Ripening fruits off the stem may then involve additional chemical exposure, fumigation, hot water, and chilling. Refrigeration of the fruit may in some cases involve weeks or months of exposure prior to its processing and shipment. Fruits may undergo additional coating with wax, coloring, or preservative films as well. Even though these treatments are intended to make the fruit taste better, they all represent forms of stress.

Yet the flavor of the fruit may conceal a hidden danger: the preternatural sweetness of these fruits may itself convey stress. The natural acquisition of sweet flavor occurs as a function of ripening, specifically as a byproduct of oxidation.

Ethylene, the stress hormone of plant life, encourages the ripening of fruits. The production of ethylene generally occurs when the plant experiences injury, dehydration, exposure to temperature extremes, or other forms of environmental stresses. In essence, the more chronic stress experienced by the plant, the more readily its fruit ripens and sweetens.

Ripening also involves increased levels of enzymatic activity. For example, apples, pears, bananas, peaches, and potatoes produce an enzyme called polyphenol oxidase. It reacts with oxygen and iron-containing phenols to produce the brownish discoloration found on the surface of these fruits. As enzymatic oxidation proceeds, the complex carbohydrates that make up the substance of the fruit also become reduced to simple sugars, which then increase the intensity of sweetness.

Simple sugars also have well-known negative effects on health. They increase the risk of tooth decay, coronary heart disease, and hypercholesterolemia (high cholesterol). They may also contribute to the development of diabetes by inducing insulin resistance and to the development of obesity by promoting the excessive intake of calories. In all of these cases, simple sugars carry an increased risk as compared to complex carbohydrates. This finding suggests that it is the message of stress carried by these simple sugars, rather than their status as carbohydrates that promotes disease.

In addition to sugars, plants can harbor stress in the form of fats. Olives and their oil offer a useful example. Integrated into the human diet for more than 5,000 years, olive oil has more recently been singled out as a critical component of the so-called Mediterranean diet that lowers the risk of heart disease, and as such has come into increasing consumer demand. Yet much of today's olive oil undergoes processing that may undermine its potential benefits to health. Small farms have traditionally made extra virgin olive oil, a designation indicating that it comes from olives picked by hand to prevent damage to skin or pulp from trees that have suffered neither disease nor drought. These olives are transported in well-aerated containers and milled within 48 hours in a single pressing to avoid oxidation. Pressing involves the time-honored use of a stone press, with the resultant olive paste further pressed by a hydraulic press without the use of heat, hot water, or solvents. The resulting oil is presented for consumption, unfiltered.

Extra virgin olive oil not only contains omega-3 fatty acids and antioxidants, both of which appear to reduce the effects of stress, but also contains oleocanthal, a compound that inhibits pathways that normally cause inflammation. In addition, recent studies have suggested that the presence of polyphenols in extra virgin olive oil appears to reduce the stress on blood vessels caused by eating fat—benefits lost with the adoption of commercial processes that increase the levels of stress exerted upon the olives. Extra virgin olive oil also may reduce the risk of many human diseases that are associated with stress. It serves as yet another example of a less stressed version of a food exhibiting fat profiles that reduce the risk of those diseases associated with stress.

Commercial production of olive oil deviates from these standards in many respects. Olives damaged from bruising or from falling to the ground are often included in the production batch, and leaves and twigs are not necessarily removed prior to milling. Transport containers lack aeration, increasing the likelihood of oxidation and mold formation. The stone press has given way to a continuous centrifuge, which uses a spinning force to separate oil from water in conjunction with heat and filtration. This process washes away the polyphenolic compounds that function as antioxidants in olives, reducing the shelf life of the oil from years to months and making it more susceptible to degradation with light exposure. Mounting evidence suggests that olive oil other than extra virgin does not confer health benefits and may indeed increase the risk of many diseases associated with stress. The stressed plants we eat may end up stressing us.

8

YOU ARE WHAT YOU EAT

So whether from flora or fauna, by land or by sea, our food supply endures a great deal of chronic stress on its journey to our plates. Still, that is no reason for it to necessarily affect our bodies in an adverse way. Yet, from the ample evidence provided by omega-6 fatty acids, saturated fats, and simple sugars, the experience of chronic stress clearly changes the composition of food. Our bodies respond to eating these foods in a manner as if we ourselves had directly undergone that stress. Further understanding as to the nature of secondhand chronic stress requires recognition as to how our bodies manage energy in the form of calories.

Our very existence requires the efficient management of energy. While we largely take in energy through the eating of food, we can use the energy we acquire in many different ways. However, how we use this energy is partly determined by our ability to forecast access to energy in the future. If we know that energy will burgeon aplenty, we will use energy more frivolously. If we know that energy will be in short supply, we will seek to conserve energy. The typical response to stress involves increased intake of food, increased storage of energy, and decreased utilization—not just in

humans, but in all organisms. Of note, physicists define stress in
denominations of energy.

In order to forecast energy availability, we must rely on hints
provided by the environment. For example, iodine can serve as a
proxy for the presence of energy. Relatively simple forms of life
such as seaweed and insects concentrate iodine as they metabolize
sources of energy, and there is evidence that they use iodine intake
to alter their metabolism. These forms of life in turn serve as dietary
staples for a variety of other organisms, ultimately dispersing iodine
throughout the food web. In humans, iodine ends up incorporated
into thyroid hormone, which controls the overall metabolic rate in
the body. With a relative absence of energy to support life, the rate
of iodine concentration throughout the food web would decline, less
iodine would end up as thyroid hormone, and the overall metabolic
rate would decrease. A relative surplus of available energy would
have an opposite effect.

A more sophisticated and sensitive measure of energy
availability would involve using the source of energy itself—
namely, food. Food possesses many qualities, such as texture,
flavor, and molecular composition, which can be defined not only in
terms of absolute quantities, but also in terms of relative amounts
and relationships to other parameters. Even given our limited
capabilities of observation and measurement, evidence shows that
the nature of food, whether as a direct product or an indirect

byproduct, clearly undergoes biochemical change in response to stress inflicted upon its source. This biochemical change is reflected in the shift from unsaturated to saturated fats, from complex carbohydrates to simple sugars, and from omega-6 to omega-3 fatty acids. Recognition of this shift may signal the relative abundance or scarcity of energy in the environment and prepare our bodies for either the bounty or the drought that lies ahead.

These examples suggest that our body uses food not only for nutrition, but also for information about the state of the environment. In a prehistoric era, the ability to forecast ecologic conditions by detecting stress in food was highly advantageous and would enhance survival. However, in the modern setting of food abundance in the developed world, our bodies' factory setting has been rendered maladaptive. The information the food chain is providing us today seems less accurate. Even though calories are abundant in the food system, we are hoarding those calories in our bodies as if winter is approaching. It does not help that modern humans are exposed to many other triggers of chronic stress such as negative news, dysfunctional human relationships, and burdensome lifestyles. The consumption of stressful information has a similar effect on our bodies as the consumption of stressed foods.

Even our taste buds may be betraying us. We postulate that our taste preferences may allow us to detect the earliest dietary signs of stress in nature. In nature, detecting ecologic stress as early as possible carries significant advantages. It enables preparation for impending challenges via conservation of resources, such as by shedding leaves in autumn or by fattening up for the winter. The exact opposite occurs at the time of the impending spring, as plants and animals alike compete to detect cues of the vernal verge, a time of increasing opportunity and abundance.

We believe that our attraction to simple sugars and saturated fats draw us to signs of stress lurking in the food web in the same way that we are drawn to car accidents and violence in the media. Simple sugars and saturated fats represent very dense sources of energy—exactly the forms of calories prized at times when the stakes for survival grow higher and more difficult.

These taste preferences may have served useful purposes in our prehistoric past, but now contribute to our poor health in the modern world. For example, the combination of sweet taste with high fat content represents a combination uncommon in nature. It comes in various guises and has become a synthetic cornerstone of many a diet—doughnuts, ice cream, cheesecake. Since sweet and fatty tastes may represent signals of stress, our bodies would then inappropriately absorb the contents of the rich meal with the gusto traditionally reserved for lean times.

Other modern methods of agriculture and husbandry may also endow food with signals of stress. Through the magic of breeding and genetic engineering, foods now yield bounty throughout the entire year—foods that in the wild would have manifested seasonality as to the time of their harvest. However, these foods may also retain signals that instruct the body to engage in a stress response mode throughout the entire year rather than in a seasonally appropriate manner. Of note, like squirrels and polar bears gorging for the harsh conditions of winter, many cultures celebrate harvest in the fall with a large feast involving sweets and fatty foods.

The more our apparent trove comes with an escalating incorporation of stress into the ways we grow, raise, and otherwise process our food, the more our bodies have become increasingly subjected to a chronic state of stress. Our bodies are responding to messages, both natural and man-made, that no longer tell the truth about how we should behave with respect to the world around us, a phenomenon we term evolutionary displacement. The notion that stressed foods are contributing to the epidemic of diseases associated with chronic stress has profound implications for our health and opens up many new avenues for medical research. We may be able to further link many other modern chronic diseases to modern changes in diet. On the other hand, we also envision a therapeutic paradigm founded on the use of low-stress foods to treat many of these same conditions.

While we await a broader movement of therapeutic foods to emerge, many food venues already offer a close approximation of what we would consider low-stress foods.

9

SOUND BITES
(SOURCES FOR LOW-STRESS FOODS)

In this section we offer a short list of vendors where consumers can currently find foods that contain less stress than foods found at most conventional establishments. This list is by no means complete, and is intended simply to serve as a starting guide. The health food movement is a moving target, but we have attempted to provide as much up-to-date information as possible. A more updated list can be found at http://www.lowstressfoods.com. We also encourage readers to visit this site to submit candidate establishments for inclusion.

SAN FRANCISCO AND THE BAY AREA

PRODUCERS:

Neff Family Ranch Natural Beef/Genesee Valley Organic Beef
4130 Genessee Rd., Taylorsville, CA
(530) 284-6371
http://www.nfrnaturalbeef.com

A 2,200-acre ranch in the Sierra Nevada Mountains of Northern California, this farm offers USDA-certified organic beef in three finishes—100% grass-fed, a balanced blend of grass and corn/grain fed, and corn/grain finished. All three types come from cattle raised as free-range their entire lives without ever seeing a feedlot—the cattle are raised on the farm's land from the time of their birth to their natural maturity. They never receive growth hormones, antibiotics or animal by-products, and eat only organic pasture, hay and grains. Skilled butchers process the cattle using hand knives rather than subjecting them to mechanical machines. Beef comes packaged either a la carte, in various combination boxes, or as a full steer or fraction thereof, including one-eighth, one-quarter, and one-half steers.

Frey Vineyards
14000 Tomki Rd., Redwood Valley, CA 95470
(707) 485-5177
http://www.freywine.com

This family-owned winery makes 100% organic wine from grapes grown using organic and biodynamic farming techniques. In addition to organic growing practices, a wine can only receive the label of "organic" if it does not contain additives such as sulfites or tartaric acid. Organic and biodynamic methods of food production seek to minimize damage to the environment and create sustainable agriculture practices. While organic growing processes indicate that the grapes are free from chemical fertilizers and pesticides, biodynamic farming also focuses on strengthening the relationships between different functional aspects of farming, such as fertility management, water management, and pest control.

Fra'Mani Handcrafted Salumi
1311 Eighth St., Berkeley, CA 94710
(510) 526-7000
http://www.framani.com

Here Paul Bertolli, the famed former chef of Berkeley's Oliveto, makes hand-crafted *salumi*—Italian-style cured or preserved meats—from high-quality, all-natural pork, in what constitutes both a wholesale and retail sausage and dry salami company. The pork comes from hogs raised on fine grains and natural feed while never receiving antibiotics, artificial growth hormones, growth-promoting agents or meat by-products. The sausages are coarse-ground, finely bound in natural hog casings, and hand-tied. The dry salami is also hand-tied with natural twine, mold-ripened, and slow-aged according to Italian tradition. Retail purchases are available online, as well as in many Bay Area markets such as Whole Foods, the Berkeley Bowl and BiRite.

Claravale Dairy
345 Kliewer Lane
Watsonville, CA 95076
(831) 722-7779
http://claravaledairy.com

This dairy farm supplies raw, completely unprocessed milk and dairy products. The pasture-grazed cows are milked by hand. The milk is then bottled immediately in glass bottles—delivered straight from the cow to the consumer. The size of their operation is very small—their milk comes from fewer than fifty Jersey cows. In addition to selling milk directly to the consumer, Bay Area Whole

Foods Markets and Rainbow Grocery stock their products, among others.

Cowgirl Creamery at Tomales Bay Foods
Ferry Building Marketplace
One Ferry Building, # 17, San Francisco, CA 94111
(415) 362-9354
80 Fourth Street, Point Reyes Station, CA 94956
(415) 663-9335
http://www.cowgirlcreamery.com

Be it the Mt Tam, a smooth, triple-cream soft cheese or the clabbered cottage cheese, many of Cowgirl Creamery's award-winning cheeses are made with organic milk from Straus Dairy, also in West Marin. The store in the Ferry Building makes it convenient to pick-up their products for a sunset snack, but can also be found in many specialty grocery shops. For a first-hand look at how things are done, you can visit the Creamery in Point Reyes Station for a tour!

Organic Pastures Dairy

7221 South Jameson Ave., Fresno, CA 93706

(559) 846-9732

http://www.organicpastures.com

Another family-owned-and-operated raw milk dairy, Organic Pastures has developed a mobile dairy barn that enables them to milk cows directly in the pasture, where the cows graze on organic grass year-round. Organic Pastures bottles its milk in plastic jugs. It offers a wide selection of other products including raw butter, raw cream, a product called Quephor™ that is similar to a drinkable yogurt, raw cheddar cheese and raw colostrums. Organic Pastures' products are available either via direct purchase or through many natural foods markets such as Whole Foods, the Berkeley Bowl, and Rainbow Grocery.

Straus Family Organic Dairy

Point Reyes, California

http://www.strausfamilycreamery.com

This family-owned dairy has pasture-grazed cows that are fed a balanced diet of organic grains, hay, legumes, home-grown silage and fresh grasses. Straus Dairy adheres to organic practices including refraining from the use of hormones or antibiotics, as well as keeping organic land and feed free from herbicides, pesticides and chemical fertilizers. While the milk is pasteurized, it is not homogenized, so the returnable old-fashioned glass bottles will need to be shaken before use. Their products are sold in grocery stores from Whole Foods and Andronico's to Rainbow Grocery across the Bay Area.

Della Fattoria
141 Petaluma Boulevard North, Petaluma, CA 94952
(707) 763-0161
http://www.dellafattoria.com
Ferry Plaza Farmer's Market and Bay Area Whole Foods

Daily, fresh-baked bread "from the farm" in Petaluma makes it to the San Francisco Ferry Plaza Farmer's Market every Saturday morning. Made from organic flour, spring water, local organic olive oil and Brittany sea salt, varieties include levain, ciabatta, Kalamata olive, seeded wheat and pumpkin seed. Della Fattoria is also available at their downtown Petaluma Café and Bay Area Whole Foods stores.

RETAILERS:

Rainbow Grocery
1745 Folsom St., San Francisco, CA 94103
(415) 863-0620
http://www.rainbowgrocery.org

An employee-owned (co-op) natural foods grocer, Rainbow Grocery
supports a standard of food production that certain farmers consider
superior to the National Organic Standards. In addition to the usual
considerations such as the avoidance of pesticide use, these farmers
take extra steps in crop rotation and maintenance of the soil so that
the growth of healthy plants do not require the addition of external
agents such as chemical fertilizers. By these measures, they hope to
institute a sustainable farming practice that should last for future
generations and have the least negative effect on the environment
and on the food.

Ferry Plaza Farmers' Market
The Ferry Building Marketplace
1 Ferry Building, San Francisco, California 94111
(415) 693-0996
http://www.ferrybuildingmarketplace.com

Locally grown fresh produce, free-range, grass-fed beef, wild caught fish, raw honey, flowers, dairy from local Cow Girl Creamery, and fresh oysters from Tomales Bay, to name just a few items—this market has it all. The Ferry Building itself houses a number of retail shops with many low-stress products ranging from wine to chocolate, in addition to restaurants that use ingredients sourced both from the market and from the local farms and vendors who come each Saturday to sell.

Planet Organics

405 Victory Ave., Unit D, South San Francisco, CA 94080

(800) 956-5855

http://www.planetorganics.com

This Bay-area based organic food home-delivery service delivers fresh produce, dairy, eggs, meat, and groceries right to your doorstep. Weekly or biweekly delivery schedules are available. Boxes of selected produce come in individual or family sizes, and assortments can be customized to taste—half vegetables and half fruits, three-quarters of one and one-quarter of the other, or all of one or the other.

Berkeley Bowl

2020 Oregon St., Berkeley, CA 94703

(510) 843-6929

http://www.berkeleybowl.com

A legendary independent supermarket, the Berkeley Bowl was started in 1977 in the former site of a bowling alley, before moving to its current 44,000 square-foot location in 1999. It is best known for its produce, to which it devotes 8,000 square feet of space. It also carries a wide variety of organic and natural foods; of particular note is an extensive section showcasing Asian foods. Also featured is a gourmet kitchen preparing a variety of traditional and exotic dishes using the freshest ingredients.

Bi-Rite Market

3639 18th St., San Francisco, CA 94110

(415) 241-9760

http://www.biritemarket.com

Specializing in sustainable artisan foods, this Mission District perennial represents a destination for restaurant-quality prepared foods, organic produce, sustainably-raised meats, poultry and seafood, as well as wine and everyday groceries. The Mogannam family has owned the market since 1964. They also maintain a family ranch from which they source fruits.

RESTAURANTS :

Boulette's Larder
Ferry Building Marketplace, San Francisco, CA 94111
(415) 399-1155
http://www.bouletteslarder.com
Chef: Amaryll Schwertner

Part marketplace, part café, and all kitchen, Boulette's Larder offers a unique perspective on the concept of take-out. A daily-changing menu offers everything needed for a full meal, or dishes to supplement a home-cooked meal. Soups, stocks, sauces, and spices are also sold. Breakfast and lunch are served Monday through Friday, and brunch is served Saturdays and Sundays. The menu features ingredients from the aforementioned Ferry Plaza Farmers' Market.

Boulevard

One Mission Street, San Francisco, CA 94105

(415) 543-6084

http://www.boulevardrestaurant.com

Chef: Nancy Oakes

Open since 1993, Chef Nancy Oakes was a James Beard Foundation winner for Best Chef in California in 2001. Mingling classic French technique with a modern, seasonal California menu, Boulevard presents a wide array of contemporary cuisine, which includes Asian, Latin and Mediterranean influences. The menu features such local delicacies as Monterey Red Abalone and California Squab.

Café Gratitude

2400 Harrison St., San Francisco, CA 94110

1336 9th Ave., San Francisco, CA 94112

1730 Shattuck Ave., Berkeley, CA 94709

2200 Fourth St., San Rafael, CA 94901

(415) 824-4652 (all locations)

http://www.cafegratitude.com

Chefs: Matthew and Terces Engelhart

Café Gratitude is an all organic, mostly raw food restaurant launched in 2004 by Matthew and Terces Engelhart, who also own a bio-sustainable, organic farm in Maui. The original intent behind the café was as a setting to play and create a community behind the "Abounding River Game," which "encourages people to be more aware and more grateful for abundance in their lives." The extensive menu consists of a wide-range of raw and/or vegan remakes of favorites such as burgers, pizza and enchiladas, in addition to salads, quinoa bowls, smoothies and desserts.

Chez Panisse
1517 Shattuck Ave., Berkeley, CA 94709
(510) 548-5525
http://www.chezpanisse.com
Chef: Alice Waters

Arguably the founder of Californian cuisine and the foremost promoter of locally grown, sustainably-harvested, organic, seasonal cooking, Alice Waters opened the doors of Chez Panisse in 1971. It soon became both an institution and a revolution. A prix-fixe set menu is served nightly in two seatings in the downstairs restaurant, and more moderately priced a la carte fare is served for both lunch and dinner in the upstairs café.

Delfina

3621 18th Street, San Francisco, CA 94110

(415) 552-4055

http://www.delfinasf.com

Chef: Craig Stoll

Fresh, local, organic ingredients come together in this popular Italian restaurant. Delfina is known for its house-cured meats and fish as well as homemade sausage, pastas and gelato. The menu features meats from Niman Ranch and Fulton Valley as well.

1550 Hyde Wine Bar and Café

1550 Hyde Street, San Francisco, CA 94109

(415) 775-1550

http://home.earthlink.net/~zootster

Chef: Peter Erickson

With its menu bearing the words, "We use local producers that practice environmentally sustainable agriculture," 1550 Hyde is known for its fresh, seasonal, organic cuisine. A café with a cozy, neighborhood feel, the menu boasts such delicious and simple dishes as balsamic marinated grass-fed skirt steak with borlotti beans, spring onion, cavolo nero and roasted garlic sauce. In addition, the extensive international wine list includes a selection of organic wines and desserts are made with dairy products from Straus Family organic dairy.

Greens
Building A, Fort Mason Center, San Francisco, CA 94123
(415) 771-6222
http://www.greensrestaurant.com
Chef: Annie Somerville

Having spearheaded standards of vegetarian cuisine nationwide in both cooking and publishing since its beginnings in the San Francisco Zen Center in 1979, Greens' purpose remains "to be of service"—by providing wholesome, seasonal vegetarian cuisine. Much of the produce comes from Green Gulch Farm in Marin and Star Route Farms in Bolinas.

Hog Island Oyster Bar
Ferry Building Marketplace
One Ferry Building, #11-1, San Francisco, CA 94111
(415) 391-7117
http://www.hogislandoysters.com

The urban extension of the Hog Island Oyster Company in the Tomales Bay Marine Sanctuary, this popular spot is famous for its fresh oysters. Favorites such as Sweetwater and Kumamotos are harvested fresh each morning and served here either raw, or in various oyster incarnations that include oysters Rockefeller, oysters casino and oyster stew. The menu also features Cowgirl Creamery grilled cheese, clam chowder and mixed green salads, as well as artisan wines and locally-brewed beers.

Jardiniere

300 Gough St., San Francisco, CA

(415) 861-5555

http://www.jardiniere.com

ACME Chophouse

24 Willie Mays Plaza, San Francisco, CA

(415) 644-0240

http://www.acmechophouse.com/

Chef: Traci Des Jardins

A post-symphony dining fixture, Jardiniere is committed to local farmers, fishers, and ranchers who use sustainable practices in growing, raising, and harvesting their products, with a particular emphasis on ocean conservation. Des Jardins is also executive chef at the ACME Chophouse, which features steaks from grass-fed cattle in addition to naturally raised poultry, local fish, and sustainable produce.

Lalime's

1329 Gilman Street, Berkeley, CA

 (510) 527-9838

http://www.lalimes.com

Fruits and vegetables are bought from local farmers markets or delivered by small local gardeners and all ingredients are chosen based on seasonality, sustainable agriculture, and fishing and farming practices. The owners, Cindy and Haig Lalime-Krikorian also host seasonal events such as a celebration marking the beginning of wild mushroom season.

Mijita

Ferry Building Marketplace

One Ferry Building, # 44, San Francisco, CA 94111

(415) 399-0814

http://mijitasf.com

Chef: Traci Des Jardins

A taqueria in the Ferry Building, Chef Traci Des Jardins of Jardiniere fame serves burritos and tacos made with Niman Ranch meats, locally caught fish and traditional Mexican cheeses, as well as the locally grown heirloom variety of pink pinto beans from Oaxaca. Organic ingredients are used whenever possible.

Millenium

580 Geary Street, San Francisco, CA 94102

(415) 345-3900

http://www.millenniumrestaurant.com

Chef: Eric Tucker

The first restaurant in the United States to offer an all-organic wine list, Millenium's vegan cuisine is made from organic, seasonal and local produce when possible and does not use any dairy or animal products in its dishes.

Modern Tea

602 Hayes St., San Francisco, CA 94102

(415) 626-5406

http://www.moderntea.com

Owner/Chef: Alice Cravens

This tea bar and café in Hayes Valley features hand-picked and hand-processed teas and herbals from organic family farms both local and abroad. Modern Tea also serves a menu of house-made soups and salads in addition to brunch offerings and classic desserts, all made from local, seasonal ingredients in cast-iron cookery. All teas are made loose leaf, and they also serve organic juices.

Oliveto

5655 College Avenue, Oakland, CA 94618

(510) 547-5356

http://www.oliveto.com

Chef: Paul Canales and Paul Bertolli

Like Chez Panisse, Oliveto is divided between an upstairs formal dining room and a downstairs café. Opened by Paul Bertolli of the new Fra'Mani Salumi venture, Oliveto strives to offer the best local, in-season, organic produce and sustainably raised meats, poultry and conscientiously harvested fish. The traditional Italian cuisine is also known for its in-house-made pasta, gnocchi, milled polenta, cured meats and sausages. There are occasional special dinners featuring particular foods such as olive oils, truffles, whole hog, spring lamb or traditional cheeses. In addition to Niman Ranch, ingredients are also sourced from such farms as the Doug Metzger Family Farm, Knoll Farms and Heritage Foods.

Pauline's Pizza

260 Valencia Street, San Francisco, CA

(415) 552-2050

http://www.paulinespizza.com

Hand-kneaded dough, Pauline's averages 150 pounds of it a day, which serves as the base for this delicious, thin-crust delight. Most of the ingredients are organic and toppings are sourced from Pauline's own Berkeley garden as well as Star Canyon Ranch. Unique toppings include Meyer lemon puree from the Meyer lemon tree in the middle of the garden, as well as home-made chicken sausage, spiced with garden-fresh herbs. Star Canyon Ranch in the Sierra Foothills supplies everything from heirloom tomatoes, to eggplant and fresh eggs that help to make the in-house desserts. In the last several years, Star Canyon Ranch has also been home to the grapes that have been turned into Pauline's Pizza Reds, a variety of wines that are featured on the menu amongst other selections from around the world. Plans for a wine bar to be opened around the corner are in the works for mid-2007.

Pizzetta 211

211 23rd Avenue, San Francisco, CA 94121

(415) 379-9880

http://www.pizzetta211.com

With a small, simple menu usually featuring five pizzas to choose from, a mixed greens salad, an artisanal cheese plate, and two delicious desserts, as well as inexpensive bottles of wine, Pizzetta 211 seats no more than 15-20 people and doesn't take reservations. The pizza dough is made fresh daily, topped with whatever is available from the local farmer's market and served until it runs out.

Rivoli Restaurant
1539 Solano Avenue, Berkeley, CA, 94707
(510) 526-2542
http://www.rivolirestaurant.com
Chef: Wendy Brucker

Rivoli features local, fresh, mostly organic cuisine that also includes sustainably caught fish and naturally raised meats and poultry. The wine list features a variety of organically raised, bio-dynamic or sustainable grown wines, which are gently handled and bottled un-fined and un-filtered.

Slanted Door
Ferry Building Marketplace
One Ferry Building, #3, San Francisco, CA 94111
(415) 861-8032
http://www.slanteddoor.com
Chef: Charles Phan

With many of the organic ingredients sourced locally right from the surrounding farmer's market, Chef Charles Phan cooks up

Vietnamese classics such as Shaking Beef using age-old traditional cooking techniques. The chicken clay pot is made with chicken from Hoffman Farms in Petaluma and a take-out version of the cuisine is available around the corner at Out the Door.

Small Shed Flatbreads
17 Madrona Street, Mill Valley, CA 94941
(415) 383-4200
http://www.smallshed.com

Situated in downtown Mill Valley, Small Shed uses only organic vegetables and grains to create its flatbreads. Featured produce comes from Star Route Farms, cheeses from Humboldt Fog and Cypress Hill and meats from the grass-fed Prather Ranch. Beverages also include organic sodas, as well as wine, beer, fresh lemonade, tea, coffee and espresso.

Tartine Bakery
600 Guerrero Street, San Francisco, CA 94110
(415) 487-2600
Bar Tartine
561 Valencia Street, San Francisco, CA 94110
(415) 487-1600
http://www.tartinebakery.com

Originally known for its bread, Tartine also offers a wide variety of pastries, tarts, cakes and cookies. All the ingredients from the flour to the sugar, herbs and fruits are organic; in addition the eggs are locally sourced and some of the cheeses come from the local Cowgirl Creamery and Cypress Grove. The wines, available by the glass and are grown organically, biodynamically or come from smaller producers in Italy and France.

Zuni Café
1658 Market St., San Francisco, CA 94102
(415) 552-2522
(no website)
Chef: Judy Rodgers

A past James Beard Foundation winner for Chef of the Year, Stanford graduate Judy Rodgers opened Zuni in 1979, and it has become one of the city's signature restaurants. Nearly all produce, meat, and fish used in the preparation of dishes have been farmed and harvested in a sustainable manner.

NEW YORK CITY

RETAILERS:

Integral Yoga
229 West 13th St., New York, NY 10011
(212) 243-2642
http://www.integralyoganaturalfoods.com

Opened more than 30 years ago in 1972 as an adjunct to the Integral Yoga Institute, this natural food store is committed to providing the highest-quality fresh, organic, vegetarian food with an emphasis on service. Over 90% of their shoppers visit the store once a week. Offerings include produce, dairy, and bulk items among others, as well as body care items and vitamins.

Green Market at Union Square
East 17th St. at Broadway, New York, NY 10003
http://www.unionsquarejournal.com/greenmarket.htm

Though there are green markets all over New York City, the largest is located at Union Square has been a fixture since 1970. It sells fresh, local, organically-grown produce, meats, dairy products, artisan breads, and fresh-cut flowers from over 200 vendors year-round, four days a week from 8 AM to 6 PM. Additional specialty items can often be found here including fresh pheasant, wild boar, and lacto-fermented products such as raw sauerkraut and ginger carrots.

Urban Organic
240 Six St., Brooklyn, NY 11215
(718) 499-4321
http://www.urbanorganic.net

Offering home delivery service of organic produce and groceries, this company makes weekly deliveries of produce available in different sized boxes. Their standard Value Box contains a variety of 15-18 different fruits and vegetables. An all-juicing produce box is also available. Delivery is free in Brooklyn and Manhattan and a small delivery fee is charged for the Outer Boroughs and New Jersey, Connecticut, Long Island, and Westchester. Additional organic grocery items include fresh-baked bread, soy products, herbs and spices, dairy products, desserts and more.

RESTAURANTS:

Pure Food and Wine
54 Irving Pl., New York, NY 10003
(212) 477-1010
http://www.purefoodandwine.com
Executive Chef: Sarma Melngalis

Pure Food and Wine is a high-end live food restaurant that uses only the freshest seasonal, organic ingredients to create live food versions of well-known favorites such as Indian samosas, tamales, and lasagna. Ice cream and other desserts are made without dairy, eggs, or sugar. Juices used in cocktails are fresh-pressed from organic fruits and are sweetened only by agave nectar, a natural, low-glycemic sweetener from the cactus plant.

Angelica Kitchen
300 East 12th St., New York, NY 10003
(212) 228-2909
http://www.angelicakitchen.com
Owner: Leslie McEachern

One of the most creative vegan restaurants in New York, Angelica Kitchen also pays special attention to ingredients sourced from responsible businesses practicing sustainable agriculture. They strive to serve food within forty-eight hours after harvest and use no refined sugars, preservatives, dairy, eggs, or animal products. They guarantee that their food is 95% grown ecologically. They deal with their purveyors, artisans, and farmers directly to ensure freshness and quality and introduce lesser-known ingredients such as sea vegetables, heirloom beans, and ancient grains to the menu when possible.

Better Burger NYC

565 Third Ave. (at 37th St.), New York, NY 10016
(212) 949-7528

178 Eighth Ave. (at 19th St.), New York, NY 10011
(212) 989-6688

587 Ninth Ave. (at 42nd St.), New York, NY 10036
(212) 629-6622

http://www.betterburgernyc.com/

The newest venture by the executive chef of Josie's, these joints offer a variety of beef, poultry, soy, and fish burgers that are antibiotic, hormone and nitrate-free, cooked in the highest quality expeller-pressed extra virgin olive and canola oils. Buns do not contain preservatives or refined sugar; organic potatoes are air-baked instead of fried; and the smoothie and drink menu offers dairy-free, organic ingredients in addition to traditional milk-based smoothies made with organic skim milk and organic yogurt.

Josie's Restaurant West

300 Amsterdam Ave., New York, NY 10023

(212) 769-1212

Josie's Restaurant East

565 Third Ave. (at 37th St.), New York, NY 10016

(212) 490-1558

Josephina

1900 Broadway, New York, NY 10023

(212) 799-1000

Citrus

320 Amsterdam Ave. (at 75th St.), New York, NY 10023

(212) 595-0500

Josie's Kitchen

1614 2nd Ave. (at 84th St.), New York, NY 10028

(212) 734-6644

http://www.josiesnyc.com

Executive Chef: Louis Lanza

With its health-conscious concept now expanded into five restaurants, the legendary Josie's focuses on dairy-free organic cuisine with an emphasis on free-range meat, poultry, eggs, and eco-friendly fish, as well as vegetarian options. The drink menu features mostly organic options including organic Rain vodka and organic wine and beer. Josephina is an upscale establishment featuring New American Cuisine. Citrus serves fusion Latin fare with an Asian flair.

Candle Café

1307 Third Avenue at 75th St.

New York, NY

(212) 472-0970

Candle 79

154 East 79th Street near Lexington

New York, NY

(212) 537-7179

http://candlecafe.com

Owners: Joy and Bart Pierson

These sister restaurants feature vegetarian cuisine using organic produce. The original Candle Café was opened in 1994 on the Upper East Side and focuses on sandwiches, salads, and wholesome entrees, while Candle 79 serves more sophisticated fare using tempeh (a whole soybean product) and seitan (wheat gluten) in place of meat.

Caravan of Dreams
405 East Sixth St., New York, NY 10009
(212) 254-1613
http://www.caravanofdreams.net

This organic vegan café is 100% kosher certified, offering both cooked and raw foods, as well as yoga and live music. Menu items include a wide variety of juices, smoothies, soups, salads, sandwiches, and snacks, in addition to vegan interpretations of Italian, Asian, Mexican, Spanish, and Middle Eastern specialties.

Cookshop
156 Tenth Ave. (at 20th St.), New York, NY 10011
(212) 924-4440
http://cookshopny.com
Executive Chef: Mark Meyers

Aiming to support local farmers and artisans as well as humanely raised animals, the Cookshop offers healthy American cuisine. The menu includes Montauk Point striped bass, Catskill duck breast, Berkshire pork chops, and Hudson Valley baby chicken and rabbit.

Souen: Organic Macrobiotic Restaurant

210 Sixth Ave. (at Prince St.), New York, NY 10014

(212) 807-7421

28 East 13th St., New York, NY 10003

(212) 627-7150

http://www.souen.net

Opened in 1971, Souen follows macrobiotic principles to offer natural, organic food with no refined, chemical, preservative, meat, or dairy ingredients. Vegetarian and fish entrees are complemented by sushi and noodle offerings.

METROPOLITAN LOS ANGELES

RESTAURANTS:

M Café Chaya

7119 Melrose Ave., Hollywood, CA 90036

(323) 525-0588

http://mcafedechaya.com

Executive Chef: Shigefumi Tachibe

M Café de Chaya provides "contemporary macrobiotic" cuisine for breakfast, lunch, and dinner to customers in this European, deli-style venue. The macrobiotic philosophy believes in achieving balance in the variety of foods eaten. M Café interprets these principles loosely to appeal to a larger audience, even extending into desserts such as chocolate cupcakes, banana bread and oatmeal raisin cookies. In addition to a wide variety of made-to-order salads, sandwiches and rice bowls, the deli case is stocked with various prepared salads and boxes to go.

Juliano's Raw
609 Broadway, Santa Monica, CA 90401
(310) 587-1552
http://www.planetraw.com
Chef/Owner: Juliano Brotman

One of the first raw and living food restaurants in the Los Angeles area, Brotman began instituting his philosophy at the first Raw in San Francisco (now closed). Dishes are made from ingredients which are organic, dairy- and animal-free, and never heated above 120 degrees.

Real Food Daily
514 Santa Monica Blvd., Santa Monica, CA 90401
(310) 451-7544
414 N. La Cienega Blvd., Los Angeles, CA 90048

(310) 289-9910
http://www.realfood.com

This is a vegan cuisine café, which means no meat, fish, fowl, dairy, eggs, butter, or animal products of any kind are used in the preparation of the food. Ingredients are never frozen, as this would destroy the cellulose in their composition, rendering them mushy and tasteless. All dishes are free of cholesterol, saturated fats, refined sugars, artificial sweeteners, white flours, preservatives, and pesticide use.

Axe
1009 Abbot Kinney Blvd., Venice, CA 90291
(310) 664-9787
http://www.axerestaurant.com
Chef/Owner: Joanna Moore

The name Axe, pronounced *ash-ay*, comes from Yoruba (now part of Nigeria) and means "go with the power of Gods and Goddesses." Axe is focused on providing simple, farm-direct, nutritious and organic cuisine in a way that encourages a feeling of community to thrive. Produce and eggs come from the Santa Monica Farmer's Market; beef is grass-fed; fish is wild; and poultry is free-range.

Providence

5955 Melrose Ave., Los Angeles, CA 90038

(323) 460-4170

http://www.providencela.com/

Chef/Owner: Michael Cimarusti

Recently named one of the fifty best restaurants in America by Gourmet Magazine, Providence features a largely seafood-based menu using only fresh, whole, natural, organic ingredients infused with vitality. Fish is either purchased from the local fish market or flown to the restaurant within 24 hours, where it is kept on ice and personally cut by the chef in a refrigerated room specially constructed for this purpose.

Inn of the Seventh Ray

128 Old Topanga Rd., Topanga, CA

(310) 455-1311

http://www.innoftheseventhray.com/

Chef: Daniel Holzman

Set in the mountains of Topanga Canyon, this former church location features outdoor seating. Most foods are organically grown and sourced from local farms. All foods are cooked in nut or olive oils; chicken is naturally raised and range-fed, with no antibiotics;

fish is fresh; and dairy ingredients are kept to a minimum. Bread is baked fresh daily with organic grains. Many wines come from small local vineyards, with some organically grown and unpasteurized.

Native Foods

The CAMP, 2937 Bristol St., Costa Mesa, CA 92626

(714) 751-2151

Westwood Village, 1110 ½ Gayley Ave., Los Angeles, CA 90025

(310) 209-1055

73-890 El Paseo, Palm Desert, CA 92260

(760) 836-9396

Smore Tree Village, 1775 E. Palm Canyon Dr., Palm Springs,

CA 92264

(760) 416-0070

http://www.nativefoods.com

CEO: Tanya Petrovna

This quartet of organic vegan and vegetarian restaurants features a wide variety of salads, sandwiches (dubbed "handholds"), hot bowls, pizza, soups, snacks, and sweets.

CHICAGO

RESTAURANTS:

Spring
2039 West North Ave., Chicago, IL 60647
(773) 395-7100
http://www.springrestaurant.net
Green Zebra
1460 West Chicago Ave., Chicago, IL 60622
(312) 243-7100
http://www.greenzebrachicago.com
Custom House
500 South Dearborn St., Chicago, IL 60686
(312) 523-0200
http://www.customhouse.cc/
Executive Chef: Shawn McClain

The 2006 James Beard Foundation award winner for Best Chef Midwest, Shawn McClain has three restaurants in Chicago. Spring focuses on seafood and other fresh, seasonal, organic ingredients that are sourced locally when possible. The cuisine is New American with strong Asian influences. The Green Zebra is a specific type of local tomato, and the second, predominantly vegetarian restaurant was so named to reflect its emphasis on use of local, regionally sourced ingredients. In contrast, Custom House places a greater emphasis on meat, including steaks and chops, as compared to the other two offerings. Nevertheless, it has not lost sight of its emphasis on sustainability.

Karyn's Fresh Corner Café
Karyn's Raw Vegan Gourmet Restaurant
Karyn's Inner Beauty Center
1901 North Halsted St., Chicago, IL 60614
(312) 255-1590
Karyn's Cooked
738 North Wells St., Chicago, IL 60610
(312) 587-1050
http://www.karynraw.com
Owner/Chef: Karyn Calabrese

Karyn's is the original raw food restaurant in Chicago. A Lincoln Park fixture, it serves vegan, raw cuisine made from whole, fresh foods that are organic whenever possible. There is no use of dairy products, eggs, refined sugar, salt, or artificial flavors. There is both a café menu and a sit-down gourmet menu offering a variety of raw foods. In addition, the recently opened Karyn's Cooked serves gourmet vegan cuisine that is not necessarily raw. While Karyn's

Raw allows you to bring your own alcoholic beverages, Karyn's
Cooked offers organic wines and beer. The restaurants are also
integrated into a spa and a retail storefront called Karyn's Inner
Beauty, which offers a variety of spa services, nutritional
consultation, and chiropractic care as well as classes and other
treatments.

Blackbird

619 West Randolph, Chicago, IL 60606

(312) 715-0708

http://www.blackbirdrestaurant.com

Executive Chef: Paul Kahan

Kahan is another former James Beard Award winner for Best Chef
in the Midwest. Located just west of the Loop, Blackbird is known
as one of the first restaurants in the area to dedicate its cuisine to the
use of specific seasonal local ingredients, putting an American touch
on French cuisine.

SEATTLE AND SURROUNDING AREAS

RETAILERS:

Pike Place Market
Parking at 1531 Western Ave., Seattle, WA 98101
http://www.pikeplacemarket.org

Established in 1907, Pike Place Market features 200 year-round commercial businesses, 190 craftspeople and 120 farmers who rent table space by the day, many of whom sell organic and sustainable offerings. It attracts 10 million visitors a year.

Pioneer Organics
901 NW 49th St., Seattle, WA 98107
(206) 632-3424
7911 NE 33rd St. Suite 220, Portland, OR 97211
(503) 460-2729
http://www.pioneerorganics.com

This home-delivery service provides local, organic, seasonal food sourced from throughout Oregon and Washington.

RESTAURANTS:

The Herb Farm

14590 NE 145th St., Woodinville, WA 98072

(425) 485-5300

http://www.theherbfarm.com

Chef: Jerry Traunfeld

Featuring cuisine made only from foods in-season from the Pacific Northwest, the restaurant grows its own herbs in the accompanying garden. Meal themes reflect the featured offerings. For example, in mid-October, A Mycologist's Dream featured wild-foraged mushrooms, collected by an in-house master wild-food forager after hundreds of miles of travel and hikes deep into the mountains. In early December, The Hunter's Table featured game of the field, winter vegetables, and wild food.

Rover's and the Chef in the Hat

2808 E. Madison St., Seattle, WA 98112

(206) 325-7442

http://www.rovers-seattle.com

Chef: Thierry Rautureau

Described by the restaurant as "Pacific Northwest cuisine with a French accent," ingredients used are local, sustainable, organic, and seasonal—bought from purveyors that include mushroom foragers, Washington State cheese makers and local farmers.

Sterling Café

2614 NE 55th St.

Seattle, WA

(206) 522-3011

http://www.sterlingcafe.net

Owner/Chef: Don Wilson

One of the first restaurants to be certified organic by the Department of Agriculture, Sterling Café offers a wide selection of meat, poultry, organic, and vegetarian dishes. All fish served are wild-caught.

WASHINGTON D.C./VIRGINIA/MARYLAND

RETAILERS:

MOM's--My Organic Market

11711 B Parklawn Dr., Rockville, MD 20852

(301) 816-4944

9827 Rhode Island Ave., College Park, MD 20740

(301) 220-1100

3831 Mt. Vernon Ave., Alexandria, VA 22305

(703) 535-5980

7351 Assateague Drive, #190, Jessup, MD 20794

(410) 799-2175

http://www.myorganicmarket.com

Supporting the environment is a top priority for this organic and natural foods market. As a component of environmental advocacy, MOM's offers a large selection of naturally and organically grown produce, products, beauty care items, and supplements. Since organic produce is stocked daily to ensure the freshest availability, MOM's doesn't open until 10 AM. MOM's also guarantees the lowest prices on all frozen, refrigerated, dry grocery, supplement, and health and beauty care products.

Door to Door Organics

7036-D Easton Rd., Pipersville, PA 18947

(888) 283-4443

http://www.doortodoororganics.com

(Serving DC, WV, VA, NY, NJ, MD, PA, DE, CT, MI, CO)

Specializing in home-delivered organic produce, Door-to-Door Organics delivers farm fresh, organic produce directly to the home. Produce can be mixed between fruit and vegetables and come in different sizes, much like the aforementioned Planet Organics.

RESTAURANTS:

Restaurant Nora

2132 Florida Ave. NW, Washington, DC 20008

(202) 462-5143

Asia Nora

2213 M St. NW, Washington, DC 20037

(202) 797-4860

http://www.noras.com

Chef/Owner: Nora Pouillon

Opened in 1979, Nora's was the first restaurant in the U.S. to be certified organic by the Department of Agriculture, and has carried this certification since 1999. This designation indicates that 95% or more of all ingredients come from certified organic growers and farmers committed to sustainable agriculture. Chef Nora Pouillon played a key role in creating this standard; only a small handful of other restaurants have ever achieved this level in the United States. The menu includes wines from small wine producers, beef reared on organic hay and cereal grains, free-range chickens, hand-made goat cheeses, fresh-picked wild mushrooms, and local Applewood smoked trout, when in season. Asia Nora shares the same fundamental values of Restaurant Nora, but offers Asian cuisine.

Sunflower
2531 Chain Bridge Rd.
Vienna, VA 22181
(703) 319-3888
http://www.crystalsunflower.com
Owners/Chefs: James and Miranda Chang

A vegetarian restaurant in suburban Northern Virginia, Sunflower's Chinese, Japanese, and continental cuisine is made from only the best quality ingredients. Many items are directly imported from their original source to ensure quality and freshness. Only organic flavor enhancers are used such as kelp powder, kombu, seal salt, gamashio, barley malt, brown rice syrup, vegetable stock, fresh nature root vegetables, and filtered water for drinking and cooking.

The Vegetable Garden
11618 Rockville Pike, Rockville, MD 20852
(301) 468-9301
http://www.thevegetablegarden.com

The Vegetable Garden offers Chinese vegetarian, vegan, and macrobiotic cuisine—some of which is certified organic, and all of which refrains from inclusion of animal products, seafood, or dairy. The restaurant also uses no monosodium glutamate in its dishes, opting instead for fresh herbs and spices. The Vegetable Garden also specifies which ingredients are organic and which are conventional in each of its dishes.

Salads and Things Organic
4213 North Fairfax Dr., Arlington, VA 22203
(703) 465-8888
http://www.saladsandthings.com

This quick-service restaurant offers soups, made-to-order salads and sandwiches, vegetarian drinks, smoothies, and teas, all from certified organic or certified all-natural farms in California, Florida, and Canada. Bread is made especially for Salads and Things by a local bakery using all-natural ingredients. They offer orders via the web, catering, take-out, and deli-style eat-in service.

NATIONAL

Whole Foods Market, Inc.
National Office:
550 Bowie Street
Austin, TX 78703
(512) 477-4455
http://www.wholefoodsmarket.com
As of February 2007: 193 locations in North America and the UK

A leader in the natural, organic grocery space, Whole Foods is committed to providing minimally processed, whole, natural foods that are free of trans-fats, artificial flavors, colors, sweeteners, and preservatives. Meat and dairy products never come from cloned animals, and are free of antibiotics and hormones. Many livestock are also grass-fed throughout their lives. Whole Foods also offers a wide variety of body care products and supplements, which adhere to the same standards as their foods.

Contrary to some claims that Whole Foods is part of the growing "industrialized organic" category, the company is positioned to make greater efforts to support local and small farm food production in the United States and throughout the world, as well as artisan food producers. The markets operate somewhat autonomously from one another with differences in product offerings based on seasonality and regional availability to ensure quality. Beginning sometime in 2007, Whole Foods will introduce its "animal compassionate" label to some of its meat and poultry products to indicate that animals were raised in a humane way. Standards include prohibiting the castration of sheep and the tail-docking of pigs, and limiting the use of electric prodding in the management of beef cattle to emergency situations. This label will go beyond the organic label, which only ensures the animals are raised without antibiotics or hormones and never fed animal by-products.

10

FOOD FOR THOUGHT

The ideas presented in this book presage a novel food system business model that can complement the existing model. In the existing model, scalable food production and distribution models generally increase stress in the underlying food. Catering to taste enhances demand and simultaneously promotes supply-chain efficiency. Competing against an extant model with such favorable economic characteristics is hardly trivial: it is reasonable to assume that low-stress foods may offer more challenging taste considerations for the consumer and a higher cost structure to the seller.

Fortunately, we now reside at a tipping point in food culture. The dialogue surrounding food has shifted from that of survival to that of health. Abundance has increasingly replaced scarcity as the dominant reality in food systems, and the negative health impact of modern foods has received an avalanche of attention. Thanks to an increased awareness of these issues, we have seen a crescendo of interest in healthy foods over time. In the presence of a perceived health benefit, a willingness to compromise a bit on taste and tolerate higher prices has emerged.

Indeed, the food industry has seized upon the obsession with health by instituting promotional campaigns that emphasize the health dimensions of the product. These tactics have usually garnered higher prices and higher margins typically associated with the premium, luxury niche. Prior blitzes have touted the salubrious qualities of oats and soy, while current efforts espouse the merits of such philosophies as organic, free-range, and probiotic. The lack of consistency in the data validating these claims reflects an incomplete understanding of the fundamental link between food and health. We believe that the stressed-food thesis presented in this book represents the common thread that mechanistically links virtually all the observed associations between food and health, particularly those involving modern food themes such as organic foods, "slow foods", raw foods, natural foods, vegetarianism, macrobiotics, local foods, and free-range meats.

The path then becomes laid for new entrants into the food industry that carry the friendly brand "low-stress foods" or its more aggressive cousin "stress-free foods". These entrants can incrementally remodel some or all aspects of production and distribution which affect the stress content of food—with the intent of promoting lower stress intake on the part of the consumer. One can envision everything from chicken farms that market their ability to sell low-stress poultry, to restaurants that offer low-stress menus.

Some existing merchants may repackage their current practices to join the brand. Others will need wholesale changes to their business models in order to fit the brand identity. Those establishments detailed in the previous chapter represent a starter list to get readers and businesses immediately engaged in the proposed movement, taking comfort in the fact that critical mass has already formed, though the movement is not currently consolidated under a well-defined, unified brand. As the brand develops and acquires premium status, the associated high margin may attract innovators who can develop new stress-relieving production and distribution methods that will further pave the way for sub-brands to emerge.

Partnership with advocacy groups, government agencies, business associations, and other stakeholders in the food culture will be critical to the success of the movement. For instance, while animal rights activists who have exposed farming practices that are stressful to animals have been successful in shaping behavioral change among some consumers, the moral arguments they employ have largely failed to sway others. Expanding the message campaign beyond the moral argument and informing the consumer about how the farming practices may directly impact their stress level may offer a powerful additional motivational tool. Resistance campaigns, especially from industry incumbents that may perceive near-term economic harm, should be anticipated and factored into the broader strategy of how to manage the movement to success. Education will need to play a key role in priming the proper motivations of various stakeholders who shape public opinion—most notably the media, and leaders in business, politics, and culture. The fundamental knowledge assets that we believe require wide promotion include (1) the notion that the body treats food as both nutrition and information about the state of the environment; (2) the idea that food can carry stress signals; (3) the concept that our body assimilates stress embedded in foods in a case of "you are what you eat"; and (4) the ways and means by which one can access low-stress foods.

Appendix 1
REFERENCES /
SOURCE MATERIALS

Due to the rapidly evolving nature of the food knowledge landscape, our list of references and source materials resides online at the website http://www.lowstressfoods.com. This bibliography reflects resources consulted for each section of the book as well as for the book as a whole. As the extent of our understanding grows, so too will this compendium.

Please visit our blog at

http://www.lowstressfoods.com/blog

Appendix 2

ABOUT THE AUTHORS / ACKNOWLEDGMENTS

Joon Yun, M.D., is a physician and a founder of the Palo Alto Institute, a non-profit think tank based out of Palo Alto, California, USA.

Stephanie Daniel is a member of the Palo Alto Institute and will be starting medical school in 2007.

Special thanks to John Doux for suggesting the word gusto.

Special thanks to Conrad Yun for his contributions to the research and editing of the book.

Special thanks to Kerry Dolan for her contributions to the positioning and writing of the book.

We would like to especially acknowledge the valuable feedback from Brian Delany, Grant Fox, Tristen Moors, and Bobby Nouredini.